Prehospital Emergency Care

A Guide for Paramedics

THIRD EDITION

Prehospital Emergency Care

A Guide for Paramedics

THIRD EDITION

Jean Abbott, M.D., F.A.C.E.P.
Assistant Professor, Emergency Medicine
University of Colorado Health Sciences Center
Denver, Colorado

Marilyn Gifford, M.D. F.A.C.E.P.
Director, Emergency Services
Memorial Hospital
Colorado Springs, Colorado

The Parthenon Publishing Group
International Publishers in Medicine, Science & Technology

NEW YORK   LONDON

Published in the USA and Canada by:
The Parthenon Publishing Group Inc.
One Blue Hill Plaza, PO Box 1564, Pearl River, NY 10965

Published in Europe by:
The Parthenon Publishing Group Ltd.
Casterton Hall, Carnforth, Lancs. LA6 2LA, UK

Library of Congress Cataloging-in-Publication Data
Prehospital Emergency Care: a guide for paramedics / Jean Abbott, Marilyn
    Gifford. -- 3rd ed.
    p. cm. -- (The Clinical handbook series)
    Rev. ed. of: Protocols for prehospital emergency medical care. 2nd ed. c1984.
    Includes bibliographical references and index.
    ISBN 1-85070-636-0
    1. Emergency medicine--Handbooks, manuals, etc. 2. Medical protocols--
    Handbooks, manuals, etc. I. Gifford, Marilyn, II. Abbott, Jean. Prehospital
    emergency care. III. Title. IV. Series.
    [DNLM: 1. Emergencies--handbooks. 2. Emergency Medical Technicians--
    handbooks. QW 52 A6313 1995]
RC86.8.A28 1996
616.02'5--dc20
DNLM/DLC
for Library of Congress   95-49532
                                                                            CIP

British Library Cataloguing in Publication Data
Abbott, Jean
Prehospital Emergency Care: a guide to paramedics. - 3rd ed. - (The Clinical
    Handbook Series)
    1. Emergency medicine 2. Assistance in emergencies
    3. Emergency medical services
    I. Title II. Gifford, Marilyn
    616'.025

ISBN 1-85070-636-0

The author has exerted every effort to ensure that drug selection
and dosage set forth in this text are in accord with current
recommendations and practice at the time of publication.
However, in view of ongoing research, changes in government
regulations, and the constant flow of information relating to drug
therapy and drug reactions, the reader is urged to check the
package insert for each drug for any change in indications and
dosage and for added warnings and precautions. This is
particularly important when the recommended agent is a new or
infrequently employed drug.

Typeset by H & H Graphics, Blackburn, UK
Printed and bound in the USA

Contents

Preface to
the Third Edition

Eleven years after publication of our Second edition, the need remains to provide active field professionals with a succinct version of the assessment and management of common problems seen in the prehospital medical arena. We have continued to actively use and modify these protocols in our own systems within Colorado. They have proven useful in many other areas of the country, so our prehospital colleagues talked us into another updated edition.

The bond between the prehospital professional and the base physician has tightened for both legal and ethical reasons. Written standards allow EMS systems to interact among each other, fire and rescue units, with specialized rescue personnel and with base stations. Written protocols allow the quality of care to be monitored regularly and facilitate the orientation of new personnel to a new prehospital management system.

The dialogue between professionals continues concerning our understanding of the correct balance between rapid transport with minimal treatment (or treatment en route) and stabilization prior to transfer, the successful cornerstone of cardiac arrest resuscitation on which the concept of prehospital care was originally based. This debate continues to alter the balance of needs. Each system needs to continue to review the much improved research literature currently ongoing so that new understandings can be incorporated into the individual modifications needed to national protocols such as these for any particular local system. Active physician participation (not only from the speciality of emergency medicine but also from trauma surgery, cardiology and other "destination" specialists), once a rarity, has become a welcome and necessary part of the dialogue about prehospital management.

The diversity of training levels, improvements in both basic and advanced equipment, and management recognition of prehospital stressors had been a healthy trend in communities. Systems have different training levels, different spectrums of illness and injury, and different capabilities at destination hospitals. This has resulted in healthy scrutiny of just which drugs and procedures are locally important, needed or possible. It does, however, make writing protocols a more dangerous and presumptive task. We have included a wider variety of drugs and procedures than many prehospital systems will want or need to use. We need, as always, to encourage prehospital systems to eliminate those parts of these protocols which are not appropriate to their system, either because of training level of prehospital providers, regional need, or the philosophy of medical direction for that region.

We continue to be deeply indebted to the American Heart Association and to the American College of Surgeons for providing leadership in standardizing early medical and trauma resuscitation algorithms. We have incorporated the latest 1994 ACLS, PALS and ATLS guidelines into our protocols with the supposition that prehospital care provides the initial steps of an integrated continuous resuscitation plan which will be carried through the emergency department, operating room, or critical care areas to provide the patient with the best possible chances for a successful outcome. The ACLS, PALS and BTLS or PHTLS courses are recommended in their entireties.

We would like to thank all of the EMTs, Paramedics and Physicians who have helped these protocols become useful tools for education, review and continuous quality improvement (CQI) activities. Thanks to Scott Smith, EMT-P for assistance with illustrations. Finally we would like to thank our offspring who were crawling when we began this endeavor and have now moved on to become EMTs, attend college, start medical school and thrive in this modern world while sharing their Moms with the prehospital environment. Thanks to Patti and Nate Abbott. Thanks to Eric and Brian Caplan.

The Authors

1

PREHOSPITAL
PATIENT ASSESSMENT

INTRODUCTION

Patient assessment in the field and in the Emergency Department is performed differently than assessment in a conventional medical setting. The routine hospital evaluation of a patient works logically through history-taking, physical examination, gathering of laboratory data, confirmation of a diagnosis, and initiation of treatment. In comparison, emergency assessment, both prehospital and in-hospital, appears disorganized. The history is often obtained after physical examination and treatment may need to be initiated before the assessment is completed. What seems disorganized should, however, be very systematic. The speed with which emergencies must be handled makes systematic assessment and care very important. Certain key questions organize the approach to emergency assessment and treatment:

1. *What is the life-threat to this patient?*

   The purpose of this primary survey is to detect life-threatening problems. Treatment of life-threats, both medical and traumatic, must be started before further assessment.

2. *What is the most serious condition that this patient could have?*

   Diagnosis of a patient in the field is often not possible. However,

1

appropriate care should be possible in most instances. It is important to treat the patient as if he or she has whatever would be most dangerous to that patient. When the patient is considered "guilty until proven innocent", the prehospital care workers are prepared for anything.

3. *What has caused the patient or family to seek help at this time?*

Particularly with medical problems, the real purpose of the call must be determined. What is new about the patient's problem? What has changed recently to make the patient or family consider this an emergency at this time?

4. *What data can be gathered from the scene that will help improve patient care?*

The EMT or Paramedic is the physician's eyes in the field. He or she is the only health-care provider who can observe the patient's environment, the mechanism of injury, empty pill bottles or syringes, and the patient's ability to care for himself. The data obtained in the field can be invaluable to patient care and outcome.

5. *How can field care keep this patient from becoming worse?*

By field stabilization, an attempt is made to prevent or minimize patient deterioration during prehospital care. Management to prevent deterioration is always a part of care, even if further treatment cannot be performed or is not indicated. Stabilization can provide relatively definitive treatment for some patients, as with splinting a fractured extremity. On the other hand, when no field techniques can keep the patient from deteriorating, treatment may consist of rapid transport to minimize time in the field.

6. *Does this patient require treatment before reaching the hospital?*

The BLS service must be aware of the transport time, the risk of delaying treatment, and the illnesses that are best managed by a call for ALS back-up or rendezvous during transport to the hospital. The ALS service must be aware of risks of treatment, expected benefits, and stability of the patient with no treatment.

7. *What treatment is appropriate for this patient?*

Some problems can be adequately documented and definitively

treated in the field (e.g., ventricular fibrillation, hypoglycemia). Some can't be diagnosed or managed in the field. Many problems lie between these two extremes. Deciding who to treat and how requires judgment:

1. How certain is the diagnosis?

2. How sick is the patient?

3. Can the problem be documented before treatment?

4. How effective is the treatment?

5. What are the hazards of the proposed treatment?

6. What are the risks of delaying treatment?

7. How much will the treatment alter the ability of the physician to assess the patient at the hospital?

8. What is the transport time?

The ability to use good judgment in assessing the patient is a more difficult and yet more valuable skill than any of the technical skills involved in prehospital treatment.

8. *Has medical authority been consulted appropriately?*

Frequently, it is necessary to make rapid assessments and treatment decisions with little time to gather information. There will always be some situations which are unclear, abnormal or complicated for many reasons. The radio is an essential tool for assessment too. Use it to share the picture with the physician or nurse. It can often lead to better understanding of the patient's illness.

9. *Have the treatment decisions taken into consideration the surroundings and the patient's situation?*

Care must be individualized. Is this patient capable of taking care of himself if he is unwilling to be transported? Is the patient competent to refuse or consent to treatment? Will the patient be *safe* if left at home or at the scene?

Patient evaluation, then, requires not just competent history-taking, or even the competent physical examination, but an evaluation of multiple factors which vary from patient to patient. Stabilization and treatment must be started without complete knowledge of what this patient's disease process may be. In addition to changes in the patient's condition, more complete information often becomes available after the initial assessment and initiation of treatment (from witnesses, newly arrived friends or relatives and other sources) requiring regular review of data and appropriate adjustments in treatment. This constantly changing set of data both limits the ability to treat in the field and provides challenge to work skillfully to make the most of field assessment with the limited tools available.

PRIMARY SURVEY: MEDICAL AND TRAUMA PATIENT

Environmental Assessment

A. Recognize environmental hazards to rescuers, and secure area for treatment. *Apply gloves and eye protection as indicated.*

B. Recognize continuing hazard for patient, and protect them from further injury.

C. Identify number of patients. Initiate a triage system if appropriate.

D. Observe position of patient, mechanism of injury, and surroundings.

E. Identify self.

F. Initiate communications if hospital resources require mobilization. Call for backup if needed.

Primary Survey

Airway, Breathing, Circulation (ABCs)

A. Airway

　1. Observe the mouth and upper airway for air movement.

　2. Open airway if needed – use head-tilt/chin-lift in medical patients, chin-lift (without head-tilt) or jaw-thrust in trauma victims.

　3. Protect cervical spine from movement in trauma victims. Use assistant to provide continuous manual stabilization (NOT traction).

　4. Look for evidence of upper airway problems such as vomitus, bleeding, or facial trauma.

　5. Clear upper airway of mechanical obstruction with finger sweep or suction as needed.

B. Breathing

　1. Expose chest and observe chest wall movement.

　2. Note respiratory rate (qualitative), noise, and effort.

　3. Treat respiratory arrest with:

　　a. Pocket mask or bag-valve-mask (BVM) for initial ventilatory control. Check pulse, begin CPR if none.

5

    b. Intubate after initial ventilations if necessary. Check tube placement.

4. Assess for partial or complete obstruction. Treat according to protocol.

5. If respiratory rate <12/minute or breathing appears inadequate:

    a. Assist respirations with pocket mask or BVM. Apply O_2.

    b. Consider tracheal intubation to secure airway if necessary. Check tube placement.

6. Observe skin color, pigmentation for signs of hypoxia. Apply O_2, high flow (10–15 L/min), by mask if signs of severe hypoxia.

7. Look for life-threatening respiratory problems and stabilize (see Chest Trauma):

    a. Open or sucking chest wound – seal.

    b. Large flail segment – stabilize.

    c. Tension pneumothorax – transport rapidly and consider decompression.

C. Circulation

1. Control hemorrhage by direct pressure with clean dressing to wound. (If needed, use elevation or pressure points. Use tourniquet ONLY in extreme situation.)

2. Palpate for radial pulse – presence implies BP > 80 systolic. If not present, check carotid or femoral pulse (presence implies BP > 60–70). If no pulses present, begin CPR.

3. Note pulse quality (strong, weak), and general rate (slow, fast, moderate).

4. If evidence of medical shock or severe hypovolemia, obtain baseline vital signs immediately and begin treatment according to protocols.

D. Responsiveness

1. Note initial level (awake, responsive to voice or pain, no response).

2. Briefly note body position and extremity movement.

Special Notes

A. Primary survey may take 30 seconds or less in a medical patient or victim of minor trauma. In the severely traumatized patient, however, assessment and treatment of life-threatening injuries evaluated in the primary survey may require rapid intervention, with treatment and further assessment enroute to the hospital.

B. In the awake patient, the primary survey may be completed by your initial greeting to the patient. This may make it clear that the ABCs are stable and emergency intervention is not required before completing assessment.

C. Neck should be immobilized and secured during airway assessment or immediately following primary survey if indicated.

D. Specific vital signs (blood pressure, pulse, respiratory rate, Glasgow Coma Score) should be obtained after the primary survey. If immediate intervention for hypoventilation or profound shock is required, this may need to be initiated before numerical vital signs are obtained.

SECONDARY SURVEY: TRAUMA PATIENT ASSESSMENT

Secondary survey is the systematic assessment of the entire patient. It should be performed after:

1. Primary survey.

2. Stabilization and initial treatment of life-threatening airway, breathing, or circulatory difficulties.

3. Cervical immobilization as needed.

4. Initial vital signs (may be done simultaneously by associate).

The purpose of the secondary survey is to uncover problems which are not life-threatening but which could be injurious or could become life-threatening to the patient.

A. Head and Face

1. Observe for deformities, asymmetry, bleeding.

2. Palpate for deformities, tenderness, crepitus.

3. Recheck airway for potential obstruction – Dentures, bleeding, loose or avulsed teeth, vomitus, abnormal tooth position from mandibular fracture, absent gag reflex.

4. Eyes – pupils (equal or unequal, shape, responsiveness to light), search for foreign bodies, or contact lenses.

5. Nose – deformity, bleeding, discharge.

6. Ears – bleeding, discharge, bruising behind ears.

B. Neck

1. Recheck manually for deformity, abrasions or tenderness if not already immobilized.

2. Observe for wounds, trauma, neck vein distention, use of neck muscles for respiration, altered voice, and medical alert tags.

3. Palpate for crepitus, tracheal shift.

C. Chest

1. Observe for wounds, symmetry of chest wall movement.

2. Palpate for tenderness, wounds, fractures, crepitus, unequal rise of chest.

3. Have patient take deep breath. Observe for pain, symmetry, air leak from wounds.

4. Auscultate for rales (wet sounds), rhonchi, wheezes, or decreased breath sounds.

D. Abdomen

1. Observe for obvious wounds, bruising, distention.

2. Palpate all four quadrants for tenderness, rigidity.

E. Pelvis

1. Palpate and compress lateral pelvic rims and symphysis pubis for tenderness or instability.

F. Shoulders/Upper Extremities

1. Observe for angulation, protruding bone ends, symmetry.

2. Palpate for tenderness, crepitus.

3. Note distal pulses, color, medical alert tags.

4. Check sensation.

5. Test for weakness if no obvious fracture, pain, or deformity present (have patient squeeze your hands).

6. If no obvious fracture, pain, or deformity gently move arms to check overall function and range of motion.

G. Lower Extremities

1. Observe for angulation, protruding bone ends, symmetry.

2. Palpate for tenderness, crepitus.

3. Note distal pulses, color.

4. Check sensation.

5. Test for weakness if no obvious fracture, pain, or deformity present (have patient push/pull feet against your hands).

6. If no obvious fracture, pain, or deformity gently move legs to check overall function and range of motion.

H. Back

1. If patient is stable – log roll, observe and palpate for wounds, fractures, tenderness, bruising.

2. Recheck motor and sensory function as appropriate.

Special Notes

A. Secondary survey should take 1–2 minutes to complete.

B. Be systematic. If you jump from one obvious injury to another, the subtle injury that is most dangerous to the patient may be easily missed.

C. Interruption of the secondary survey should only occur if the patient experiences airway, breathing or circulatory deterioration. Otherwise complete the survey *before* beginning to address the secondary problems that have been identified.

D. Auscultate chest either during the secondary survey or after the survey is completed and the stethoscope is out for vital signs.

E. Obtain and record two or more sets of vital signs and neurologic observations prior to transport or en route. A patient cannot be called "stable" without at least two sets of vital signs giving similar "normal" readings.

F. Orthostatic vital signs are of questionable value. Physiologic variability is great, and a barely compensated patient with hypovolemia can be made critical by the stress of upright or even sitting position.

G. The concept of "stable" probably has no place in the field evaluation of the trauma patient. Patients with apparently "normal" vital signs in the field can "CRASH" in the emergency department – not due to inadequate evaluation – but because their normal body compensatory mechanisms become overwhelmed. Occult hemorrhage is difficult to detect without specialized studies. It may first be suspected when the patient develops signs of shock. At that point the blood loss may be close to lethal. (The only truly "stable" trauma patient is the one you cared for yesterday and who is now under observation and doing well.)

PATIENT HISTORY: MEDICAL AND TRAUMA PATIENT

Medical

A. Chief complaint

1. When did it start? How long has it been going on? Is it changing?

2. How intense is the problem? Very severe, mild?

3. What caused or brought on the condition?

4. Does anything make it better or worse?

5. For pain – describe the location, type of pain, severity, radiation.

6. What caused the patient or family to seek help at this time?

7. Has the patient experienced or been treated before for this problem? When? What was the usual treatment?

8. Are any other symptoms bothering the patient at this time?

B. Associated complaints – Question as for chief complaint.

C. Relevant past medical history.

D. Allergies.

E. Medications and drugs – Chronic and "on-board".

F. Survey of surroundings for evidence of drug abuse, mental functioning, family problems.

Trauma

A. Chief complaints – Areas of tenderness, pain.

B. Associated complaints – Trouble breathing, dizziness.

C. Mechanism of injury

1. What were the implements involved – weapons, autos, machinery?

2. How did the injury happen – cause, precipitating factors?

3. What trajectories were involved – bullets, cars, people?

4. How forceful was the mechanism – speed of cars, force of blow, height of fall?

    5. With a vehicle – What is the condition of windshield, steering wheel, body? Were the passengers wearing seatbelts?

D. Mental status and pertinent findings since accident according to witnesses or bystanders.

E. Treatment since accident – Movement of patient by bystanders, etc.

Special Notes

A. Do not let information gathering distract from the management of life-threatening problems.

B. Appropriate questioning can provide valuable information while establishing authority, competence, and rapport with patient.

C. Two types of information are used to assess medical or trauma conditions. Subjective information is related by the patient in taking a history, and describes *symptoms*. The physical exam provides *signs*, or objective information, which may or may not correlate with the patient's symptoms.

D. In medical situations, history is commonly obtained before or during physical assessment. In trauma cases it may be simultaneous or following the secondary survey. An assistant is often used for gathering information from patient or bystanders.

E. In trauma cases, carefully examine all areas where the patient complains of pain, but realize that the patient's capacity to feel pain is usually limited to one or two areas – even if more are injured! Patients under the influence of drugs or alcohol may not feel pain in spite of significant injuries. That is why a systematic survey is important even in an awake patient.

F. Use bystanders to confirm information obtained from the patient and to provide facts when the patient cannot. History from the scene is invaluable.

G. Over-the-counter medications (including aspirin and "cold remedies") are frequently overlooked by patient and rescuer, but may be important to emergency problems.

SECONDARY SURVEY: MEDICAL PATIENT ASSESSMENT

A primary survey is done on all medical and trauma patients. In awake medical patients, this may consist only of identifying yourself and noting the patient's responsiveness and general appearance. A full head-to-toe secondary survey may not need to be done on patients with a specific complaint, such as "chest pain". Assessment must be no less thorough, but it may be limited to the body systems that are pertinent to the presenting problem.

A. Vital signs – Quantitative vital signs usually precede the rest of the exam.

B. Head/Face

    1. Note airway patency, oral swelling, hydration.

    2. Eyes – note pupil symmetry, reaction to light, movement.

    3. Note symmetry of facial movements.

C. Neck

    1. Observe for neck vein distention in the upright position, use of accessory muscles for breathing.

D. Chest

    1. Observe chest wall for symmetry of air movement and evidence of respiratory effort.

    2. Auscultate:

        a. Breath sounds for symmetry, rales (wet sounds), wheezing, or evidence of obstruction.

        b. Heart for regularity (if irregular, is it intermittently or consistently irregular?).

E. Abdomen

    1. Observe for distention, bruising.

    2. Palpate (gently) for tenderness, rigidity, masses.

F. Extremities

    1. Observe – presence of edema, color of skin.

    2. Palpate for warmth, tenderness, presence of pulses, capillary refill.

G. Neurologic exam – See Neurologic Assessment.

PEDIATRIC PATIENT ASSESSMENT

Children can be examined easily from one end to the other, but lack of understanding by the patient, poor cooperation, and fright often limit the ability to assess completely in the field. The "Head-to-Toe" approach in children probably needs to be a "Toe-to-Head" approach. The exam needs to be systematic, but if the primary survey does not reveal immediate life threats, the child will be less threatened by a more distant approach to begin the exam. Observations about spontaneous movements of the patient and areas that the child protects are very important.

A. Primary Survey

   1. Airway, Breathing, and Circulation.

   2. Evaluate and secure.

B. General

   1. Level of alertness, eye contact, attention to surroundings.

   2. Muscle tone – normal, increased, or weak and flaccid.

   3. Observe responsiveness to parents, caregivers. Is the patient playful or irritable?

C. Extremities

   1. Brachial pulse.

   2. Signs of trauma.

   3. Muscle tone, symmetry of movement.

   4. Skin temperature and color, capillary refill.

   5. Areas of tenderness, guarding or limited movement.

D. Abdomen – Observe child for bruises, abrasions, distention, rigidity, or tenderness.

E. Chest

   1. Note presence of stridor, retractions (depressions between ribs on inspiration) or increased respiratory effort. Respiratory rate.

   2. Breath sounds – symmetrical, wet, wheezing?

   3. Heart – rate, obvious murmur.

F. Neck – Note stiffness.

G. Head

    1. Signs of trauma.

    2. Fontanelle, if open – abnormal depression or bulging.

H. Face

    1. Pupils – size, shape, symmetry, reaction to light.

    2. Hydration – brightness of eyes. Is the child making tears? Is the mouth moist?

I. Neurologic Assessment – see page 16.

TABLE 1-1. NORMAL VITAL SIGNS IN THE PEDIATRIC AGE GROUP

Age	Pulse beats/min	Respirations rate/min	Blood Pressure systolic +/–20
Premature	144	20 – 38	N/A
Newborn	140	20 – 38	N/A
6 mo	130	20 – 30	80 palp
1 yr	125	20 – 24	90 palp
3 yr	110	20 – 24	95 palp
5 yr	100	20 – 24	95 palp
8–10 yr	90	12 – 20	100 palp

NEUROLOGIC ASSESSMENT

Management of patients with head injury or neurologic illness depends on careful assessment of neurologic function. *Changes* are particularly important. The first observations of neurologic status in the field provide the basis for monitoring sequential changes. It is therefore important that the first responder accurately observe and record neurologic assessment, using measures which will be followed throughout the patient's hospital course.

A. Vital Signs – Observe particularly for adequacy of ventilations, depth, frequency, and regularity of respirations.

B. Level of consciousness

Glasgow Coma Score

Eye opening:	None	1
	To pain	2
	To speech	3
	Spontaneously	4
Best verbal response:	None	1
	Garbled sounds	2
	Inappropriate words	3
	Disoriented sentences	4
	Oriented	5
Best motor response:	None	1
	Abnormal extension	2
	Abnormal flexion	3
	Withdrawal to pain	4
	Localizes pain	5
	Obeys commands	6

Glasgow coma score = Sum of scores in
  3 categories:
  (15 points possible)

C. Eyes

  1. Direction of gaze.

  2. Tracking of gaze.

  3. Size and reactivity of pupils.

D. Movement – Observe whether all four extremities move equally well, have equal strength.

E. Sensation (if patient awake) – Observe for absent, abnormal or normal sensation at different levels if cord injury is suspected.

Special Notes

A. The Glasgow Coma Scale (GCS) is one method of scoring and monitoring patients with head injury. It is readily learned, has little observer-to-observer variability, and reflects cerebral function. Always record specific responses rather than just the score (sum of observations). In areas where numerical assignment of scores is not a formal procedure, the observations of the coma scale still provide an excellent basis for field neurologic assessment. The other parameters listed must be observed to fully assess the impaired patient.

B. Use a flow sheet to follow and identify changes.

C. Sensory and motor exam must be documented before moving patient with suspected spinal injury.

D. Sensory deficit levels should be marked gently on the patient's skin with a pen to help identify any changes.

E. Note what stimulus is being used when recording responses. Applied noxious stimuli must be adequate to the task but not excessive. Initial mild stimuli can include light pinch, dull pinprick, or light sternal rub. If these are unsuccessful at eliciting a pain response stronger pinch (particularly in axilla), or sternal rub will be necessary to demonstrate the patient's *best* motor response.

F. When responses are not symmetrical, use motor response of the best side for scoring GCS and note asymmetry as part of neurologic evaluation.

G. Use of restraints or intubation of patient will make some observations less accurate. Note on chart if circumstances do not permit full verbal or motor evaluation.

H. In small children, the GCS may be difficult or impossible to evaluate. Children who are alert and appropriate should focus their eyes and follow your actions, respond to parents or caregivers, and use language and behavior appropriate to their age level. In addition, they should have normal muscle tone and a normal cry.

I. Drug ingestion, hypotension, and alcohol intoxication can all depress the GCS. Since the effects of drugs or alcohol cannot be assessed in the field, the score may be depressed for reasons other than head injury. The GCS cannot, therefore, be used for prognostication. It's main contribution is to monitor deterioration or improvement of the patient.

TRIAGE: MULTIPLE PATIENT ASSESSMENT

Definition   Triage, from the French – to sort, sift or pick out. Specifically, the sorting of and allocation of treatment to patients.

Indications   Medical (usually traumatic) emergency involving more than one patient, interaction between different agencies, and the need to make choices regarding treatment.

Priorities

A. Park vehicle in safe location.

B. Do initial assessment of scene. Proceed only when safe to rescuer.

C. Rapidly estimate number of victims and severity of injuries *(Do not provide treatment)*.

D. Establish communications and request necessary assistance. Provide initial estimate of number and types of injuries. Notify hospitals.

E. Designate or ensure designation of:

   1. Medical command – the person with the most medical training and experience. That person should:

     a. Coordinate medical resources with patient needs. Maintain communications with involved agencies.

     b. Select stabilization area which is safe, close, and has good access for drive-through of multiple emergency vehicles.

     c. Appoint triage team if not already organized.

     d. Select recorder to assist with written log of patients – age, sex, category and where transported.

     e. Direct, with Incident Command (overall scene commander), flow of ambulances to and from scene.

     f. Oversee patient flow to ambulances and hospitals such that:

       1. Critical patients are transported first when possible.

       2. Distribution of critical patients to hospitals is balanced with bed supply and hospital resources.

2. Triage team:

   a. Categorize and tag patients after brief assessment.

   b. Update categorizations and provide transport to stabilization area as able.

   c. Initiate medical stabilization to patients awaiting transport after triage duties completed.

3. Transport team (if necessary):

   a. Transport patients in order of priority from field to stabilization area.

   b. Establish IVs or perform other stabilization procedures as needed in support of triage team.

Precautions

A. Identification of medical charge personnel is extremely important and often overlooked. Use vests, hats, or other labeled equipment. Keep a kit in each vehicle.

B. Location of stabilization area is very important. It should fulfill the following criteria:

   1. Away from objective dangers of scene.

   2. Close enough for access from scene for stretchers.

   3. Accessible by multiple rescue vehicles, both in and out.

   4. Near communications and other command personnel for coordination of evacuation.

C. Attach triage tags to patient, not clothing. Triage tags should be uniform in each region so they are readily recognized by all responders. There should be a way to record vital signs, findings, problems list, medications given, etc. on the tags. The tags should also reflect the status of the patients.

> Red – I – Critical; requiring care within 30–60 minutes.
> Yellow – II – Urgent; care within 60–120 minutes.
> Green – III – Delayed; care within 12 hours.
> Black – IV – Dead (or near dead).

D. Triage assessment and management differs from single patient assessment. Certain problems recur in major disasters and should be avoided:

  1. Do not use up ambulance space initially transporting "green" patients before more serious injuries have been transported.

  2. Do not delay transport to treat patients at the scene.

  3. Reassess patients when able and correct tags to reflect your new assessment. Triage is a continuous process.

  4. Disaster scenes may have many talented medical persons; only one can be "Chief". Be sure that person is well-identified, and be a good "Indian" if that is your role.

Special Notes
A. Multiple-patient scenes will always be a challenge to prehospital planning and ingenuity. Disaster drills *can* be very worthwhile and practice *does* help. Small simulations involving 6–10 patients often teach much to the segment of the system doing the exercise, and allow more frequent practice for "the big one".

B. A "mini-disaster" plan which allows appropriate mobilization of extra personnel to accommodate 6–10 patients without unnecessarily activating large numbers of people is very useful. This can be coordinated both within a hospital or within a region for more efficient back-up when resources are stretched.

C. The Incident Command (IC) structure developed and disseminated by the National Interagency Incident Management System (NIIMS) and Federal Emergency Management Agency (FEMA) provides an excellent overall approach to disaster management. The structure is designed to allow flexibility and local differences, as well as incorporate different training levels (physician, nurse, paramedic, EMT) within medical control at the scene.

D. Multiple-trauma patients with no vital signs on arrival of rescue personnel have a *very* poor chance of survival even if they are the only victim. If there are additional victims with any signs of life, attention will be better spent with the living.

TRIAGE DECISION SCHEME

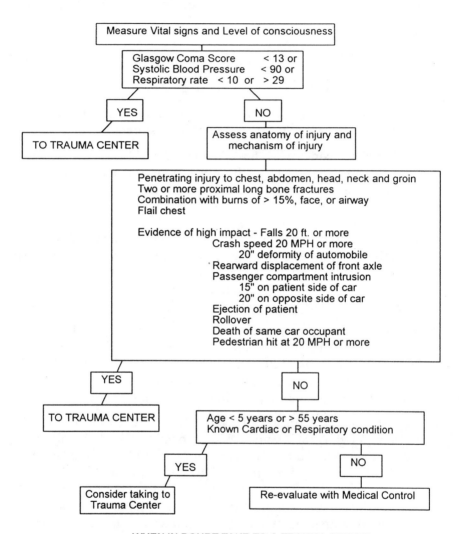

Measure Vital signs and Level of consciousness

Glasgow Coma Score   < 13 or
Systolic Blood Pressure   < 90 or
Respiratory rate   < 10   or   > 29

YES → TO TRAUMA CENTER

NO → Assess anatomy of injury and mechanism of injury

Penetrating injury to chest, abdomen, head, neck and groin
Two or more proximal long bone fractures
Combination with burns of > 15%, face, or airway
Flail chest

Evidence of high impact - Falls 20 ft. or more
       Crash speed 20 MPH or more
       20" deformity of automobile
       Rearward displacement of front axle
       Passenger compartment intrusion
       15" on patient side of car
       20" on opposite side of car
       Ejection of patient
       Rollover
       Death of same car occupant
       Pedestrian hit at 20 MPH or more

YES → TO TRAUMA CENTER

NO → Age < 5 years or > 55 years
Known Cardiac or Respiratory condition

YES → Consider taking to Trauma Center

NO → Re-evaluate with Medical Control

WHEN IN DOUBT TAKE TO A TRAUMA CENTER

(American College of Surgeons, Committee on Trauma, Resource document)

22

DEATH IN THE FIELD

Indications

I. Pronouncement of death in the field (without initiation of resuscitation) should include the following instances:

Patient unresponsive, apneic, pulseless, *and* with

A. Decapitation, or

B. Decomposition, or

C. Rigor mortis with warm air temperature, or

D. Multiple casualty situation where system resources are required for stabilization of living patients, or

E. Advanced Directive which specifies *do not resuscitate.*

II. Certain other circumstances may require exception and personnel should receive permission from base physician (with BLS in progress) at the time of the occurrence:

Patient unresponsive, apneic, pulseless, *and* with

A. Advanced age, showing extreme wasting of severe chronic disease, or

B. Pre-arranged written "no resuscitation" order for terminal patient by patient's physician, or

C. A verbal "no resuscitation" order from an attending physician who is present at the time. This physician should be able to identify him/her self and provide information about the patient consistent with an ongoing relationship. A physician who "drops by" to help and has no knowledge of the patient is *not* considered an attending physician, or

D. A verbal "no resuscitation" order from an attending physician via radio or phone. If at all possible these physicians should be requested to contact the emergency physician at the base or receiving hospital to clarify the course of action.

Precautions

A. Death cannot be judged in the hypothermic patient who may be asystolic, apneic, and stiff but may still survive intact. Transport for rewarming in all instances.

B. Those who fall under the guidelines in I. (decapitation, decomposition, etc.) should be left at the scene with law enforcement personnel. Many children will still be transported to the emergency department, as parents will frequently bring them out to the transporting vehicle. The grief of pediatric death is sometimes better managed at the hospital. However, with police chaplains or crisis response teams, the family may receive adequate support at home. An added benefit of allowing the family to grieve in their home is that no "false hopes" will be raised by overly aggressive prehospital care.

C. Do not attempt to guess future outcomes based on appearance of the patient (e.g., shotgun blast to face of suicide victim). Failure to act because of mistaken notions of outcome will be a self-fulfilling prophecy.

D. Do not allow suicide to prejudice the decision to resuscitate. No matter how psychiatrically serious, a patient may, after therapy, resume the desire to live. It is inappropriate to agree with the patient that death would be preferable, and therefore fail to act.

E. Do not delay action to find out facts about patient's history. If summoned, one must respond. If the patient has a chronic disease (for instance, cancer), the place to educate relatives as to the inevitability of death (if indeed that is appropriate) is at the hospital, not in the field.

F. Even with "Do Not Resuscitate" orders, if there seems to be any disagreement among the family, it is better to err on the side of *providing* life support. That may not apply to Advanced Directives which are specific indications of the patient's wishes. Generally these directives will carry the force of law. Check with State EMS Divisions for specific state guidelines.

Special Notes

A. Be careful to avoid discussion of the mechanism of death in the presence of relatives. In early grief, it is easy to misinterpret even well meaning expressions of concern. Moreover, because a patient is doing well in the field does not mean that survival is assured. Misguided optimism in the field will make grieving more difficult later.

B. Rescue personnel, like emergency department personnel, must have the ability to discuss their own grief over problem cases with each other and their advisers. Moreover, they must come to terms with their mission, what can be accomplished in the field (not every life can be saved), and the importance of having resolved ethical issues before taking care of individual problems.

C. When you, as an EMS responder, are summoned, you should initiate resuscitation. In these days when we are becoming more concerned with the right to die with dignity, do not allow premature judgment to delay or withhold life-saving skills. Despite much press to the contrary, BLS and even ALS measures are extremely unlikely to "bring back" an otherwise unsalvageable person.

D. Drowning patients with submersion less than 60 minutes in cold water; patients with hypothermia; or patients who are pregnant and believed to be 20 weeks or later in gestation should receive full resuscitative efforts since there are occasionally "miraculous" recoveries.

E. If the situation appears to be a potential crime scene, EMS providers should disturb the scene as little as possible.

2

MEDICAL TREATMENT PROTOCOLS

INTRODUCTION TO TREATMENT PROTOCOLS

The following five chapters contain recommended treatment protocols for common presenting prehospital problems. The problems are divided into the following categories:

Chapter 2:   Medical
Chapter 3:   Pediatric Medical
Chapter 4:   Trauma
Chapter 5:   Environmental
Chapter 6:   Hazardous Materials

Within each chapter, the problems are organized in alphabetical order.

We have attempted to present the problems wherever possible by the presenting symptoms or findings, rather than by the diagnosis. Patients rarely present with a known diagnosis, and often field diagnosis is neither necessary nor desirable. The decisions about when and how to treat must be based on data available to the EMT or Paramedic at the scene. We have tried to apply this principle whenever possible.

Each protocol is organized according to the history (specific information needed), physical findings (specific objective findings), treatment steps, and specific precautions. The treatment steps contain some starred (*) medications. These are medications which are appropriate to advanced personnel only with direct physician orders. Non-starred items are appropriate for advanced personnel by standing order administration, without necessity of direct verbal physician order. Paramedics should also feel free to initiate direct radio contact for standing order drugs in cases where the diagnosis is unclear or the protocol does not seem appropriate.

The choice of which medications to stock, which to allow by standing order, and which procedures to utilize, should be made by the medical director in conjunction with the emergency care community.

ABDOMINAL PAIN

Specific information needed

A. Pain – nature (sharp, dull, crampy, constant or intermittent), duration, location; radiation to back, groin, chest, shoulder.

B. Associated symptoms – nausea, vomiting (bloody or coffee-ground), diarrhea, constipation, black or tarry stools, urinary difficulties, menstrual history, fever.

C. Past history – previous trauma, abnormal ingestion, medications, known diseases, surgery.

Specific objective findings

A. Vital signs.

B. General appearance – restless, quiet, sweaty, pale.

C. Abdomen – tenderness, guarding, bowel sounds, distention, pulsatile mass.

D. Emesis – appearance, amount.

Treatment

A. Position of comfort.

B. NPO.

C. O_2, moderate flow (4–6 L/min). Titrate to pulse oximetry > 90%.

D. If BP < 90 systolic and signs of hypovolemic shock:

    1. Increase O_2, high flow (10–15 L/min). Titrate to pulse oximetry > 90%, if possible.

    2. Apply PASG and inflate per protocol.

    3. IV – volume expander (NS or RL), large bore, TKO or as directed.

E. IV, volume expander (NS or RL), TKO if vital signs normal but pain severe and transport time > 15 minutes.

F. Monitor vital signs during transport.

Specific precautions

A. Causes of abdominal pain can rarely be determined in the field. Pain medication is seldom indicated and may change details of the physical exam necessary to diagnose the patient in the emergency department.

B. The most important diagnoses to consider are those associated with catastrophic internal bleeding: ruptured aneurysm, liver, spleen, ectopic pregnancy, etc. Since the bleeding is not apparent, you must *think* of the volume depletion and monitor patient closely to recognize shock.

C. Elderly patients may have significant hypovolemic shock with systolic blood pressures above 90 mm Hg. With signs of hypovolemia (see medical shock) contact base and treat with fluids and PASG as above.

D. Deep palpation, or overly aggressive testing for areas of pain is inappropriate and may actually be dangerous. Gentle palpation or testing for subtle rebound by abdominal wall percussion provide a more realistic evaluation of abdominal tenderness (and do not risk *causing* the abdominal tenderness by your exam.)

E. Recent studies on shock with continuing blood loss (such as intra-abdominal bleeding) suggest the patient may do better without rapid fluid replacement before the bleeding is stopped. Attempting to titrate blood pressure in the field is obviously not practical, but attempts to return the blood pressure to "normal" may not improve the patient's chance for survival and may increase their internal bleeding.

F. Upper abdominal and lower chest pain may be due to intrathoracic problems such as MI, dissecting aneurysm, etc. Large fluid boluses may be contraindicated. Contact base for discussion.

ALLERGY/ANAPHYLAXIS

Specific information needed
A. History – exposure to allergens (bee stings, drugs, nuts, seafood most common), prior allergic reactions.

B. Current Symptoms – itching, wheezing, respiratory distress, nausea, weakness.

C. Medications.

Specific objective findings
A. Vital signs, level of consciousness.

B. Respiration – wheezing, upper airway noise, effort.

C. Mouth – tongue or upper airway swelling.

D. Skin – hives, swelling, flushing.

Treatment
A. Ensure airway, suction as needed.

   Early intubation may be advisable before swelling becomes severe.

B. Position of comfort (upright if respiratory distress predominates, supine with PASG if shock prominent).

C. O_2, high flow (10–15 L/min), by reservoir mask if respiratory distress severe. Titrate to pulse oximetry > 90% if possible.

D. Remove injection mechanism if still present (stinger, needle, etc.).

E. If signs of severe generalized reaction are present:

   1. IV – volume expander (NS or RL), large bore, TKO.

   2. *Diphenhydramine 50 mg IV.

F. If BP < 90 systolic and signs of shock: *(Anaphylaxis)*

   1. Fluid bolus – 20 ml/kg, volume expander (NS or RL) IV.

   2. Apply PASG, inflate if systolic BP < 90 and titrate to patient condition.

   3. *Epinephrine 1:10,000, 1 ml slow IV in adult.

   4. *Diphenhydramine 50 mg IV.

31

    5. *May repeat epinephrine dose once after 5 minutes if needed.

G. For respiratory distress:

    1. Albuterol 2.5 mg/3 ml by nebulization. May need to repeat or give constant nebulizations with severe wheezing.

    2. *Epinephrine, 1:1,000, 0.3 ml SQ in adult (0.01 ml/kg SQ in child)

       Use SQ dose if patient BP > 90 systolic. (Use IV dose as above if patient hypotensive.)

    3. *Diphenhydramine 50 mg IV if needed.

H. Monitor cardiac rhythm in all patients who require treatment.

I. Transport rapidly if patient unstable. Call for back-up if needed. Prepare to assist ventilations if respiratory arrest occurs.

Specific precautions

A. Allergic reactions can take multiple forms. Early consultation with base physician is encouraged.

B. Anxiety, tremor, palpitations, tachycardia, and headache are not uncommon with administration of epinephrine. These may be particularly severe when epinephrine is given IV. In children, epinephrine may induce vomiting. In elderly patients, angina, MI or dysrhythmias may be precipitated.

C. Two forms of epinephrine are carried as part of paramedic equipment. The standard ampules of aqueous epinephrine contain a 1:1,000 dilution appropriate for SQ or IM injection. IV epinephrine should be given in a 1:10,000 dilution. Use the "cardiac" epinephrine which is premixed for IV dosing to avoid mistakes. *Be sure you are giving the proper dilution to your patient.*

D. Before treating anaphylaxis, be sure your patient has objective signs as well as subjective symptoms. Patients who are hyperventilating will occasionally think they are having an allergic reaction. Epinephrine will just aggravate their anxiety.

E. Lethal edema may be localized to the tongue, uvula or other parts of the upper airway and restrict air flow. Examine closely, and be prepared for early intubation before swelling compromises airway.

ALTERED MENTAL STATES/BEHAVIORAL PROBLEMS

Specific information needed

A. History – recent crisis, physical or emotional trauma, bizarre or abrupt changes in behavior, suicidal ideation, alcohol/drug intoxication, toxic exposure, exertion or heat exposure.

B. Past history – previous psychiatric disorders, medical problems (seizures, diabetes) or medications (including insulin, anti-depressants, other mood-altering drugs).

Specific objective findings

A. Vital signs (note pupil size, symmetry, reactivity).

B. Mental status – see Neurologic Assessment.

C. Characteristic odor to breath.

D. Medical alert tags.

E. Outside air temperature; patient's temperature.

Treatment

A. Ensure airway, breathing, and circulation.

B. *Remove or have police remove dangerous objects (e.g., weapons, drugs).*

C. Consider hyperthermia or hypothermia, and treat according to protocols.

D. Restrain *if necessary* (lateral recumbent position preferred).

E. *Consider administration of droperidol 0.1 mg/kg IV or IM if patient is so violently combative that restraint or provision of medical care endangers personnel or patient.

F. Do not leave patient unattended.

G. Explain all procedures to the patient and try to establish rapport.

H. If patient is not alert or vitals unstable:

1. Start O_2, high flow (10–15 L/min). Titrate to pulse oximetry > 90% if possible.

2. IV – volume expander (NS or RL), large bore, TKO or as directed.

3. Test blood for glucose level.

4. Administer dextrose 50%, 50 ml, IV in secure vein if glucose level < 60 mg/dl and patient unable to take sugar orally.

5. Consider naloxone, 2 mg IV for suspected narcotic toxicity.

I. Transport in calm, quiet manner, monitoring vital signs en route.

Specific precautions

A. It is important not to forget the organic causes for altered mental states. Psychiatric disorder must be at the bottom of your list, or you may forget important, treatable conditions.

Hypoxia	Postictal states
Hypoglycemia	Drug exposure/overdose
Head injury	Toxic/inhalant exposure
Hyperthermia	Hypothermia
Shock (hypovolemia, anaphylaxis)	

B. An odor of alcohol is very common in emergency patients, and often is not the primary problem. Do not blame the alcohol without looking carefully first for other potential problems.

C. If the patient is medically stable and emergency treatment is not needed, do not unnecessarily invade the patient's privacy. Try not to escalate verbal violence to physical violence. Do not shout at or ridicule your patient.

D. If the situation appears threatening, a show of force involving police may be necessary before an attempt to restrain the patient is made. Consider your own safety and limitations. Use enough back-up to be confident and forthright. The use of droperidol to assist with potentially or actually violent patients is also not without risk. When used properly, however, it should increase the safety of both patient and health care providers. Remember to allow sufficient time for the IM injection to take effect before attempts to transport a difficult patient. If patient needs to be subdued for the injection – restraint should probably be maintained until transported.

E. Beware of the combative patient who becomes quiet. Check vital signs and airway promptly, and begin resuscitation if needed. Conversely, some patients may regain consciousness due to resuscitation, and then pull out IVs or ET tubes. Be alert!

CARDIAC ARREST

Specific information needed
A. History of arrest – onset, preceding symptoms, bystander CPR, or other treatment; duration of arrest.

B. Past history – disease, medications.

C. Surroundings – evidence of drug ingestion, trauma, other unusual presentations.

Specific objective findings
A. Absence of consciousness.

B. Terminal or no respirations.

C. Absence of pulse.

D. Signs of trauma, blood loss.

E. Air temperature, skin temperature.

Treatment
A. Check surroundings for safety to rescuers.

B. Transfer to a firm surface.

C. Initiate CPR.

D. Call for back-up if needed.

E. Check rhythm with monitor or quick look paddles.

F. Treat according to rhythm – see appropriate table.

Specific precautions
A. Cardiac arrest in a trauma situation is not treated according to this protocol. In a trauma situation, transport should be rapid, with IV, PASG, CPR en route. In prolonged transport situations, or with the agreement of the EMS system, blunt trauma patients found to be in full cardiac arrest, who are unresponsive to airway maneuvers, may be left at the scene for the coroner (See Special Trauma Problems).

B. Survival from cardiac arrest is related to the time to *both* BLS and ALS treatment. Don't forget CPR in the rush for advanced equipment. A call for back-up should be initiated promptly by any

BLS unit. Likewise, standing order administration of the first steps in treatment is recommended to minimize time delays to ALS.

C. See Neonatal and Infant/Child Resuscitation Protocols for special pediatric details.

D. Large peripheral veins (antecubital or external jugular) are preferred IV sites in an arrest.

E. Quick-look paddles are preferred for initial rhythm check. Change to patches for more secure reading. Be sure machine is set to record from whichever mode is in use.

F. Be sure to recheck for pulselessness and unresponsiveness upon arrival, even if CPR is in progress. This will avoid needless and dangerous treatment of "collapsed" patients who are inaccurately diagnosed initially or who have spontaneous return of cardiac function after a dysrhythmia or vasovagal episode.

G. Do not disconnect an AED which has not completed the sequence of shocks. After the first three shocks, care may be transferred to an arriving ALS company.

TABLE 2-1. VENTRICULAR FIBRILLATION
PULSELESS VENTRICULAR TACHYCARDIA

A. Check for responsiveness, respiration, pulse.
B. Initiate CPR until defibrillator set up.
C. Confirm rhythm by monitor or quick-look paddles.
D. Defibrillate at 200 joules.
E. If no response, immediately recharge and again defibrillate at 200–300 joules.
F. If no response, immediately recharge, defibrillate at 360 joules.
G. If no response: Resume CPR.
    1. Intubate, oxygenate, control ventilation
    2. IV – NS, TKO.
H. Epinephrine, (1 mg) 10 ml, 1:10,000 IV or (2.5 mg) 2.5 ml of 1:1000 diluted with NS via endotracheal tube. (Repeat IV dose every 3–5 minutes.)
I. Defibrillate at 360 joules 30–60 seconds after epinephrine.
J. Lidocaine, 1.5 mg/kg IV – CPR for one minute.
K. Defibrillate at 360 joules.
L. Bretylium, 5 mg/kg IV – CPR for one minute.
M. Defibrillate at 360 joules.
N. Magnesium sulfate 2 gm IV – CPR for one minute.
O. Defibrillate at 360 joules.
P. Sodium bicarbonate, 1 mEq/kg, IV, if 10 minutes have elapsed without conversion – CPR for one minute.
Q. Contact base and prepare for transport.

When rhythm restored:

A. Check pulse. Treat pulseless rhythm as PEA, if pulse > 60 administer lidocaine, 1.5 mg/kg IV bolus repeat in 3–5 minutes to total of 3 mg/kg.
B. Treat dysrhythmias according to protocol if persistent.
C. *Consider dopamine or epinephrine drip to treat hypotension if it persists for > 5 minutes after conversion.

Special note: Do not overreact to varying dysrhythmias which predictably occur directly after defibrillation. Monitor pulses and blood pressure. Give the patient a chance to stabilize.

Standing orders should expediate care – not prolong scene time. Rapid transport is still the goal!

TABLE 2-2. AUTOMATIC EXTERNAL DEFIBRILLATION

A. Check for responsiveness, respirations, pulse. Call for ALS.
B. Initiate CPR.
C. Attach AED to patient. Analyze rhythm.
D. If NO SHOCK INDICATED, check pulse, continue CPR, apply oxygen, reanalyze after one minute if NO SHOCK INDICATED transport patient and continue to reanalyze every 1–2 minutes.
E. If shock indicated, defibrillate at 200 joules.
F. Analyze rhythm – if indicated – defibrillate at 200–300 joules.
G. Analyze rhythm – if indicated – defibrillate at 360 joules.
H. If no pulse:
   1. Resume CPR, and continue for 1–2 minutes.
   2. Control airway by best technique available. Administer oxygen, high flow.
I. Analyze rhythm – if indicated – defibrillate at 360 joules.
J. Recheck pulse. Continue CPR if no pulse, and transport patient.
K. Contact base to advise status.
L. When rhythm restored: check for pulse. Check vital signs, and re-institute CPR if vital signs are lost.
M. If ventricular fibrillation or tachycardia returns, repeat defibrillation with 200 joules (as in E). Repeat through H as needed.
N. If AED is in analyze/shock process when paramedics arrive wait through one sequence without disruption before changing to more advanced monitor /defibrillator.

Note: Do not be overly concerned with the many dysrhythmias that normally occur immediately after successful defibrillation. With good oxygenation and ventilation, the patient often stabilizes over the transport time.

This defibrillation protocol is for specially trained EMTs who have been individually approved by their physician advisor for this procedure.

TABLE 2-3. ASYSTOLE

A. Check for responsiveness, respirations, pulse.
B. Initiate CPR.
C. Confirm asystole. Check lead placement connections. Observe for deflection with CPR to confirm monitor function.
D. Intubate, oxygenate, and control ventilation.
E. IV – NS, TKO.
F. Confirm asystole in at least 2 leads.
G. Consider possible causes:
    1. Hypoxia.
    2. Hyperkalemia or hypokalemia.
    3. Preexisting acidosis.
    4. Drug overdose.
    5. Hypothermia.
H. Consider transcutaneous pacing.
I. Epinephrine, (1 mg) 1:10,000, 10 ml IV or (2.5 mg) 1:1000, 2.5 ml diluted with NS via ET. Repeat IV dose every 3–5 minutes as needed.
J. Atropine, 1 mg IV or 2 mg via ET.
K. Consider sodium bicarbonate, 1 mEq/kg, IV for prolonged down time or suspected hyperkalemia or tricyclic antidepressant toxicity.
L. Monitor rhythm – if unchanged, continue CPR, contact the resource hospital and discuss transport orders or consider terminating efforts.

TABLE 2-4. PULSELESS ELECTRICAL ACTIVITY

A. Check for responsiveness, respiration, pulse.
B. Initiate CPR.
C. Confirm rhythm by monitor or quick-look paddles.
D. Intubate, oxygenate, control ventilation.
E. IV – volume expander (NS or RL), wide open, 20 ml/kg if hypovolemia suspected.
F. Consider non-cardiac causes for PEA and treat:
  1. Hypovolemia: PASG and volume load.
  2. Hypoxia: Oxygen and ventilation.
  3. Pericardial tamponade/rupture: volume load and rapid transport.
  4. Tension pneumothorax (detectable with increased difficulty bagging patient): needle decompression.
  5. Hypothermia: CPR, ventilatory assist, rapid transport for rewarming.
  6. Pulmonary embolus: vigorous CPR and rapid transport.
  7. Drug overdoses such as tricyclic antidepressants: Sodium bicarbonate.
  8. Hyperkalemia, acidosis: Sodium bicarbonate.
G. Epinephrine, (1 mg) 1:10,000 10 ml IV or (2.5 mg) 1:1000, 2.5 ml diluted with NS via ET. Repeat IV dose every 3–5 minutes as needed.
H. Check for carotid or femoral pulses at least every 5 minutes, continue CPR if needed.
I. Atropine 1.0 mg IV if bradycardic (< 60/minute). Repeat 1.0 mg IV in 3 minutes if rate < 60/minute.
J. Consider sodium bicarbonate, 1 mEq/kg IV if long down time, or suspected hyperkalemia or tricyclic antidepressant toxicity.
K. Prepare for transport. Contact base hospital for further orders or consultation.

Special notes:
A. The reversible causes for PEA are noncardiac, and should be considered early.
B. Treatment of PEA assumes that the cardiac rate is adequate (> 60). Treat the rate first if the patient is bradycardic.
C. *Standing orders should expedite care – not prolong scene time. Rapid transport is still the goal.*

CHEST PAIN

Specific information needed
A. Pain – nature, severity, duration, location, onset, radiation, aggravation, alleviation, relationship to exertion.

B. Associated symptoms – nausea, vomiting, diaphoresis, respiratory difficulty, cough, fever.

C. Past history – previous cardiac or pulmonary problems, medications, drug allergies.

Specific objective findings
A. Vital signs.

B. General appearance – color, apprehension, sweating.

C. Signs of heart failure – neck vein distention, peripheral edema, respiratory distress.

D. Lung exam by auscultation – rales, crackles, wheezes, or decreased sounds.

E. Chest wall tenderness, abdominal tenderness.

Treatment
A. Reassure and place patient at rest, position of comfort.

B. O_2, moderate flow (4–6 L/min). Titrate to pulse oximetry > 90%.

C. If patient's history suggests a cardiac origin to the chest pain:

1. Monitor cardiac rhythm.

2. Obtain 12 lead EKG if equipment is available – transmit to hospital if possible.

3. IV – Saline lock, NS or RL, TKO.

4. Normalize pulse by treating tachycardia > 150 or bradycardia < 60 according to protocols.

5. Administer nitroglycerin, 0.4 mg (1/150 grain) SL, if blood pressure > 90 systolic. *Repeat every 5 minutes (x3) or until pain relieved or systolic BP < 90.

6. Administer lidocaine if PVCs > 6/minute, multiform or runs present:

41

    a.   Lidocaine bolus, 1 mg/kg body weight slow IV push.

    b.   *Consider lidocaine drip, 1 gm in 250 ml D5W. Begin administration at 2 mg/min (30 microdrops/min).

    c.   *Consider 2nd bolus of lidocaine (0.5 mg/kg) IV, 10 minutes after first bolus. Repeat to total of 3 mg/kg.

    d.   *Consider magnesium sulfate, 1–2 gm IV over 15 minutes.

7. *Administer morphine sulfate, 2–4 mg IV (repeated every 5 minutes, if indicated; but not to exceed 0.2 mg/kg) if pain persists after second nitroglycerin and BP > 100 systolic.

8. Consider the risks and benefits of thrombolytics. Notify the ED of potential AMI patient to prepare for possible thrombolysis.

D. If patient's condition is stable, transport promptly without use of lights or siren.

E. Monitor cardiac rhythm and vitals en route.

Specific precautions

A. Suspicion of an acute MI is based on history. Do *not* be reassured by a "normal" monitor strip. Conversely, "abnormal" strips (particularly ST and T changes) can be due to technical factors or nonacute cardiac diseases. ST elevation that changes after nitroglycerin administration can be significant. Changes should be documented and relayed to physician on arrival at ED.

B. Constant monitoring is essential. As many as 50% of patients with acute MIs who develop ventricular fibrillation may have no warning dysrhythmias.

C. Lidocaine should not be given if:

    –   Blood pressure < 90 systolic, or

    –   Heart rate < 60/minute, or

    –   Periods of sinus arrest or any A-V block are present, or

    –   Patient rhythm is atrial fibrillation.

D. If patient develops depressed respirations following morphine sulfate administration, be prepared to actively support airway and ventilations.

E. Consider causes other than cardiac for chest pain – pulmonary embolus, dissecting aneurysm, pneumothorax, pneumonitis, etc.

F. Be particularly cautious to avoid excessive fluids in cardiac patients.

CHILDBIRTH

Specific information needed
A. History of pregnancy(s) – due date (EDC), bleeding, swelling of face or extremities, prior problems with pregnancy, prenatal care.

B. Current problems – if pain, where? Regular? Timing? Ruptured membranes? Vaginal fluid drainage? Urge to push?

C. Medical history – medications, medical problems, patient's age, number of prior pregnancies, allergies.

Specific objective findings
A. Vital signs, particularly any degree of hypertension.

B. Swelling of face or extremities.

C. Contraction and relaxation of uterus.

D. Where privacy is possible, examine perineum for:

   1. Vaginal bleeding or fluid – Color? Odor?

   2. Crowning (head visible during contraction)?

   3. Abnormal presentation (foot, arm, cord)?

E. If delivery occurs, APGAR score of child (1, 5, and 10 minutes after delivery).

Treatment
A. If not pushing or bleeding, transport, position of comfort, avoid supine position.

B. If bleeding is moderate to heavy:

   1. O_2, moderate flow (4–6 L/min). Titrate to pulse oximetry > 90%

   2. IV – volume expander (NS or RL), large bore, TKO or as directed.

C. Transport immediately – previous cesarean section, multiple births, abnormal presenting part, excess bleeding.

D. If question of imminent delivery, observe for 1 or 2 contractions, then transport unless delivery is in progress. Be prepared to stop ambulance if delivery occurs en route.

E. If delivering:

1. Use clean or sterile technique.

2. Guide and control but do not retard or hasten delivery.

3. Suction mouth (Figure 2-1) (to back of mouth only, not throat), then nose with bulb syringe after head is delivered. Endotracheal suction is preferred with meconium stained amniotic fluid. Keep infant level with perineum.

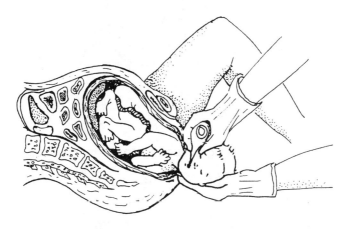

Figure 2-1. Initial suctioning

4. Suction again after delivery. Stimulate by drying. Keep warm.

5. Observe infant:

    a. If color poor, child limp, or poor vital signs (APGAR 7 or less), see Neonatal Resuscitation.

    b. If child pink, crying and moving well (APGAR 8–10), dry completely, wrap in clean or sterile dry blanket, and place next to mother to conserve heat.

6. Clamp cord in two places 8–10 inches from infant.

7. Cut cord between clamps (Figure 2-2); give infant to mother and allow to nurse to aid in uterine contraction.

8. IV – volume expander (NS or RL), large bore, TKO.

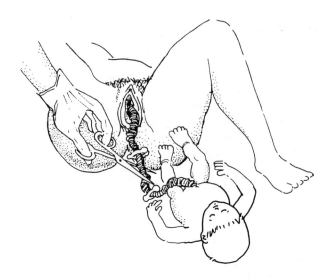

Figure 2-2. Cutting the cord

9. If excessive bleeding occurs postpartum:

    a. Massage uterus gently.

    b. Apply PASG; inflate legs per protocol.

    c. Administer IV fluid bolus, 20 ml/kg.

    d. *Consider oxytocin 20–40 mg in 500 ml NS or RL.

10. Transport. Do not wait for or attempt delivery of placenta. If placenta delivers spontaneously, take it to the hospital for inspection. Monitor vitals during transport.

Specific precautions

A. It is safe to assume that any medical or trauma condition will be complicated by pregnancy. Conversely, pregnancy can be complicated by any trauma or medical condition. The abdominal pain complained of by a pregnant woman *may not be uterine contractions.* Consider other problems.

B. Do not pull on cord. Premature delivery of the placenta is accompanied by tearing, partial separation, and occasionally severe bleeding.

C. Patient with prolapsed cord should be placed in left lateral recumbent position in Trendelenburg. The knee-chest position is generally described as the preferred position, but seems difficult to perform safely in a moving vehicle. If adequate restraints are available to *comfortably* and *safely* restrain, knee-chest may be preferred. Gloved hand may be used to keep presenting part of infant from impinging on the cord (in either position).

D. Eclampsia may complicate any pregnancy. Hypertension (often of mild degree) and peripheral edema are usually evident, and the patient may exhibit behavior changes or muscle irritability. Seizures occurring before or after the time of delivery may cause hypoxic risk to fetus or mother. Keep diazepam handy in case seizures occur, but do not administer prophylactically. Magnesium sulfate may be ordered for hypertension and/or seizures.

E. Supine hypotension occurs after 20 weeks in some women, due to compression of the Inferior Vena Cava by the gravid uterus. The left lateral recumbent position is optimum for avoiding this.

F. *Ask* patient if she feels as though she's delivering. Particularly with prior deliveries, most mothers will know. Subsequent deliveries are frequently faster.

G. Babies are slippery. It is considered poor form to drop one.

H. The outside world is cold! Babies have poor temperature regulation and no clothes. Bundle, preferably with mother. It will make them both feel better.

I. Keep your cool. Women have been delivering babies for many years. In most cases you will do nothing more than preside at a natural event.

COMA

Specific information needed

A. Present history – duration of illness, onset and progression of present state; antecedent symptoms such as headaches, seizures, confusion, or trauma.

B. Past history – previous medical or psychiatric problems.

C. Medications – use or abuse.

D. Surroundings – check for pill bottles, syringes, etc, and bring with patient. Note odor in house, general condition of house.

Specific objective findings

A. Safety to rescuer – check for gases or other toxins.

B. Vital signs.

C. Level of consciousness and neurological status.

D. Signs of trauma – head, body.

E. Breath odor.

F. Needle tracks.

G. Medical alert tag.

Treatment

A. Airway – protect as needed with positioning, NP or OP airways, suctioning, intubation.

B. O_2, high flow (10–15 L/min). Titrate to pulse oximetry > 90% if possible.

C. IV – volume expander (NS or RL), TKO or as directed.

D. Test blood for glucose level.

E. Administer dextrose 50%, 50 ml IV, in secure vein, if glucose level < 60 mg/dl.

F. Administer naloxone 2 mg IV for suspected narcotic toxicity.

G. Monitor cardiac rhythm.

H. Transport in lateral recumbent position. (If trauma suspected, supine with cervical collar and backboard; log roll as necessary.)

I. Monitor vitals during transport.

Specific precautions

A. Be particularly attentive to airway. Difficulty with secretions, vomiting, and inadequate tidal volume are common.

B. Hypoglycemia may present as focal neurologic deficit or coma (stroke-like picture) in elderly persons.

C. Coma in the diabetic may be due to hypoglycemia or to hyperglycemia (diabetic ketoacidosis). Dextrose should be given to all unconscious diabetics, as well as patients with coma of unknown origin unless a reading in the high range is obtained. The treatment may be life-saving in hypoglycemia, and will usually do no harm in the normal or hyperglycemic patient. Do not give oral sugar to an unconscious patient.

D. Although dextrose will usually do no harm, *hyper*glycemia may aggravate cerebral edema in a patient with a cerebral vascular accident. This is the primary reason to recommend that blood sugar always be determined prior to administration of glucose.

E. Naloxone is useful in any potential overdose situation, but be sure the airway and the patient are controlled before giving naloxone to a known drug addict. The acute withdrawal precipitated in an addict may result in violent combativeness. It is sometimes preferable to intubate and support, rather than to awaken the patient.

DYSRHYTHMIAS: GENERAL

Specific information needed
A. Present symptoms – sudden or gradual onset, palpitations.
B. Associated symptoms – chest pain, dizziness or fainting, trouble breathing, abdominal pain, fever.
C. Prior history – angina, dysrhythmias, cardiac disease, exercise level, pacemaker.
D. Current medications, particularly cardiac.

Specific objective findings
A. Vital signs.
B. Signs of poor cardiac output:
   1. Altered level of consciousness.
   2. "Shocky" appearance – cold clammy skin, pallor.
   3. Blood pressure < 90 systolic.
C. Signs of cardiac failure (increased back-up pressure):
   1. Neck vein distention.
   2. Lung congestion, crackles (rales).
   3. Peripheral edema – sign of chronic failure, not acute.
D. Signs of hypovolemia:
   1. Sinus tachycardia, 100–150 (usually).
   2. Flat neck veins.
   3. Poor peripheral perfusion.
   4. Evidence of blood loss (see Medical Shock.)
   5. Evidence of dehydration (dry mouth, tenting skin, etc.)
E. Signs of hypoxia: marked respiratory distress, cyanosis, tachycardia.
F. Signs of hypothermia: cold skin, decreased level of consciousness.

Treatment
A. O_2, high flow (10–15 L/min). Titrate to pulse oximetry > 90% if possible. Place in position of comfort.

B. IV – NS, TKO.

C. Evaluate the patient: *Is the patient perfusing adequately or are there signs of inadequate perfusion?*

D. Apply cardiac monitor and evaluate rhythm:

1. Is there a pulse corresponding to the monitor rhythm?

2. Rate – tachycardia, bradycardia, normal?

3. Are the ventricular complexes wide or narrow?

4. What is the relationship between atrial activity (P waves) and ventricular activity (QRS-T complexes)?

5. *Is the dysrhythmia potentially dangerous electrically to the patient?* (See Note D. below.)

E. Document the rhythm by paper tape recording or telemetry.

F. Treat if needed according to pulse rate (see protocols) or as directed by base physician.

G. Document results of treatment (or lack thereof) by checking pulse and recording change on paper tape or telemetry.

H. Transport non-emergency if patient is stable. Monitor condition en route.

Specific precautions

A. *Treat the patient not the dysrhythmia!* If the patient is perfusing adequately, he does not need emergency treatment. This is true of bradyrhythms as well as tachyrhythms. What is normal for one person may be fatal to another.

B. Documentation of dysrhythmias is extremely important. Field treatment of a dysrhythmia may be life-saving, but long-term treatment requires knowing what the problem was. Documentation also allows for learning and discussion after the case. These cases are not common, and should be reviewed and used as learning tools by as many prehospital personnel as possible.

C. Correct dysrhythmia diagnosis based only on monitor strip recordings is difficult and often not possible. Treatment must be based on observable parameters: rate, patient condition and distance from the hospital. Whenever possible, treatment in the field should be undertaken only after consultation with base physician.

D. Electrically "dangerous" rhythms are those which do not necessarily cause poor perfusion, but are likely to deteriorate. They require recognition and treatment to prevent degeneration to mechanically significant dysrhythmias. Among the electrically dangerous rhythms are: multiple and multifocal PVCs, ventricular tachycardia, and Mobitz II 2nd degree block.

E. Cardiac arrest and life-threatening dysrhythmias can be successfully treated in the field, and show the benefits of "stabilization prior to transport" in prehospital care. The patient is better off when the duration of arrest or poor perfusion is minimized.

DYSRHYTHMIAS: TACHYCARDIA

Rhythm strip assessment
A. Rate, regularity of complexes.

B. Ventricular complexes – wide (QRS > .12) or narrow.

C. P waves if detectable and relation to QRS.

Indications for treatment
A. Signs of poor perfusion – BP < 90 systolic, diaphoresis, confusion, dizziness.

B. Chest pain.

C. Signs of hypovolemia (poor perfusion plus low venous pressure).

D. Pulmonary edema.

Treatment
A. O$_2$, high flow (10–15 L/min). Titrate to pulse oximetry > 90% if possible.

B. IV – volume expander (NS or RL) TKO or as directed.

C. If pulse >100 and < 150, look for signs of hypovolemia and treat according to Medical Shock Protocol.

D. *Narrow complex* tachycardia, *regular* rhythm, pulse > 150:

    1. Good perfusion – observe.

    2. Conscious but signs of poor perfusion:

        a. Consider Valsalva and observe monitor for gradual or abrupt slowing.

        b. *Consider carotid sinus massage.

        c. *Consider adenosine 6 mg IV rapid push.

        d. *Contact base to discuss further options such as use of sedation, *cardioversion, repeat *adenosine or *verapamil if indicated.

    3. Unconscious:

        a. *Cardiovert at 100 joules on synch.

    b. *If no *discharge*, repeat at 100 joules unsynchronized.

    c. *If no *conversion*, repeat at 200 joules.

E. *Narrow complex* tachycardia, *irregular* rhythm pulse > 150:

    1. Good perfusion – observe.

    2. Conscious but signs of poor perfusion or unconscious – *cardiovert, as above.

F. *Wide complex* tachycardia, pulse > 150:

    1. Good perfusion:

        a. *Lidocaine, 1 mg/kg, IV.

        b. If no response – observe, transport.

    2. Conscious but signs of poor perfusion:

        a. *Lidocaine, 1 mg/kg, IV.

        b. *Repeat lidocaine, 0.5 mg/kg IV every 5 minutes to total 3 mg/kg if rhythm unchanged.

        c. *Adenosine, 6 mg rapid IV push.

        d. *Consider bretylium 5 mg/kg administered over 8–10 minutes if dysrhythmia persists.

        e. *Consider magnesium sulfate, 1–2 gm IV over 15 minutes.

        f. *Consider sedation with diazepam 5–10 mg IV prior to cardioversion.

        g. *Cardiovert, as previously.

        h. *Contact base to consider: further cardioversion, or additional medication administration.

    3. Unconscious with ventricular rate > 150:

        a. *Cardiovert at 100 joules on synch.

        b. *If no response, defibrillate at 200 joules; if no response, continue with Cardiac Arrest Protocol.

        c. *After conversion, administer lidocaine, 1 mg/kg IV, followed by drip. Second bolus after 10 minutes.

Specific precautions

A. Wide complex tachycardias may be ventricular or supraventricular in origin. Treatment should be based on adequacy of perfusion. Assume ventricular tachycardia in the emergency care setting if the patient is symptomatic.

B. It is most difficult to know how aggressive to be in treating the patient in the "grey" zone: symptomatic but conscious. Discuss with base, consider transport time, patient complaints, and vital signs.

C. Tachycardia is most likely a secondary problem with rate variation over time or when the pulse < 150. Treat hypoxia, hypovolemia, pain and other problems first.

D. Unconscious patients (from CVA or other causes) may present with a secondary tachycardia. Unconsciousness due to the tachycardia is usually associated with a rate greater than 180 and poor peripheral pulses.

DYSRHYTHMIAS: NORMAL RATE

Rhythm strip assessment
A. Rate.

B. Regularity, evidence of atrial fibrillation, A-V block.

C. P waves – relationship to ventricular complexes.

D. Ectopic beats – wide or narrow?

Indications for treatment
A. Premature wide complex beats (presumed PVCs) *in presence of chest pain* which occur:

    1. > 6 per minute.

    2. Multiformed.

    3. Couplets or in runs.

    4. Closely coupled (QR/QT less than 0.85)

B. Relative contraindication to treatment:

    Atrial fibrillation, hypotension, age greater than 70 years, or conduction blocks.

Treatment
If no pulse, initiate CPR and treat according to PEA protocol. Otherwise:

A. O_2, high flow (10–15 L/min). Titrate to pulse oximetry > 90% if possible.

B. Patient in position of comfort.

C. Apply monitor.

D. IV, volume expander (NS or RL), TKO or as directed.

E. If BP < 90 systolic – treat for Shock, Medical

F. If BP > 90, determine if atrial fibrillation or any conduction block exists (lst, 2nd, or 3rd degree). If so, avoid treatment and discuss options with base.

G. If BP > 90 and patient in normal sinus rhythm, treat significant PVCs in presence of chest pain with:

1. Lidocaine 1 mg/kg IV, *followed by 2–4 mg/min infusion; may administer 0.5 mg/kg IV after 10 minutes.

2. Administer nitroglycerin, 0.4 mg, SL. *Repeat after 5 minutes if no response.

3. *Consider magnesium sulfate, 1–2 gm IV over 15 minutes.

4. *Administer morphine sulfate, 2–4 mg IV (repeated every 5 minutes if indicated, but not to exceed 0.2 mg/kg). Use if pain persists after second nitroglycerin and BP > 100 systolic.

H. Contact base to consider lidocaine for PVCs in absence of chest pain.

I. Monitor patients with conduction block closely to detect deterioration of rhythm.

Specific precautions

A. PVCs are common in elderly patients who are seen for any reason. They should only be treated in the presence of acute cardiac symptoms. Discuss any other indications with base before treatment.

B. Atrial fibrillation is commonly complicated by wide complex beats. Many of these are not ventricular, despite their looks. In addition, lidocaine can cause uncontrolled ventricular rates. Avoid treatment when not essential.

C. Propranolol and other beta-blockers can prevent the tachycardic response to pain, hypoxia, or hypovolemia. Look carefully for hidden problems in patients on these medications.

D. Acute atrial fibrillation may cause hypotension because the atrial "kick" is lost and ventricular filling suddenly becomes less adequate. Acutely, it is usually accompanied by a ventricular response > 150/minute. If the ventricular rate is in the normal range, the rhythm is most likely chronic. Look for other causes of patient deterioration.

DYSRHYTHMIAS: BRADYCARDIA

Rhythm strip assessment
A. Rate.

B. Relation of P waves to ventricular complexes.

C. Irregular ventricular complexes (block or atrial fibrillation)?

D. Ectopic beats – premature or late?

Indications for treatment
A. Signs of poor perfusion – BP < 90 systolic, diaphoresis, dizziness, confusion, chest pain.

B. Pulse < 60 in patient > 40 years old.

C. Presence of premature ventricular contractions or ventricular escape beats.

D. Relative contraindication to aggressive treatment – atrial fibrillation.

Treatment
A. O_2, high flow (10–15 L/min). Titrate to pulse oximetry > 90% if possible.

B. Patient in position of comfort.

C. Apply monitor.

D. IV – volume expander (NS or RL), TKO.

E. *Atropine, 0.5 mg, IV if signs of poor perfusion. May repeat every 3–5 minutes if needed to total of 2 mg or 0.04 mg/kg.

F. *Consider dopamine, 5 to 20 mcg/kg/min IV drip, starting at 5 mcg/kg/min. Increase as needed to reach pulse > 60 or BP > 90 systolic.

G. *Prepare transcutaneous pacer for third degree block or Mobitz II, second degree block. *Consider sedation with diazepam.

H. *Consider epinephrine drip 2 to 10 mcg/min if above unsuccessful.

I. Consider options with base physician and transport rapidly if transvenous pacemaker indicated.

J. If pulses disappear, initiate CPR and treat as PEA.

Specific precautions

A. If patient in atrial fibrillation, do not use atropine or dopamine unless absolutely necessary (to avoid provoking uncontrolled ventricular response).

B. Pain from injury can occasionally cause marked vagal stimulation, with bradycardia and hypotension. This will respond to positioning with legs elevated or administration of atropine or fluids. Pain control may also be helpful.

C. Well conditioned athletes may normally be bradycardic, with pulses equal to or less than 40 beats/minute; ask your patient what is normal for him or her. In the setting of chest pain or possible acute MI, sinus bradycardia under 60 beats/minute should be treated when it is associated with hypotension or ectopy.

D. Second or third degree heart block should not be treated if the patient is doing well. Chronic 3rd degree block is often well tolerated, particularly when the ventricular rate is 50 or above. Symptoms most often occur when the block develops acutely.

E. Differentiate premature ventricular beats from escape beats, which are wide complexes occurring *late* after the preceding beat as a lower pacemaker cell takes over. Escape beats are beneficial to the patient and should be treated by increasing the underlying rate and conduction, not by suppressing the escape beat. Premature beats associated with a bradycardia also may respond to increasing rate, but at times may need to be treated with lidocaine.

HYPERTENSION

Specific information needed
A. History of hypertension and current medications.

B. New symptoms – dizziness, nausea, confusion, visual impairment, paresthesias, weakness.

C. Drug use – phenylpropanolamine, amphetamines, cocaine.

D. Other symptoms – chest pain, breathing difficulty, abdominal/back pain, severe headache.

Specific objective findings
A. Evidence of encephalopathy – confusion, seizures, coma, vomiting.

B. Presence of associated findings – pulmonary edema, neurologic signs, neck stiffness, unequal peripheral pulses.

C. Diastolic pressure > 120.

Treatment
A. O$_2$, moderate flow (4–6 L/min). Titrate to pulse oximetry > 90%.

B. Place patient supine or at rest in position of comfort.

C. Recheck BP, with special attention to diastolic pressure, correct cuff size and placement.

D. Treat chest pain, pulmonary edema, or seizure activity as per usual protocols.

E. IV – Saline lock or D5W, TKO.

F. If diastolic remains at or above 120 on repeated readings *and* patient has symptoms of encephalopathy, chest pain, or pulmonary edema, consider:

    1. *Nitroglycerin, 0.4 mg SL and repeat every 3 minutes until diastolic pressure < 100.

    2. *Morphine sulfate, 2–4 mg IV; may repeat every 3 minutes to total 0.2 mg/kg.

    3. *Furosemide, 20–40 mg IV.

G. Monitor cardiac rhythm.

H. Monitor vital signs and mental status during transport.

Specific precautions

A. Secondary hypertension (high BP in response to stress or pain) is commonly seen in the field. It does not require field treatment, and may not even mean the patient has chronic hypertension requiring ongoing treatment.

B. Hypertensive encephalopathy is rare, but can be treated if present with sedation, nitroglycerin, morphine and furosemide. Hypertension is more common in association with other problems (pulmonary edema, seizures, chest pain, coma, drug use/abuse or altered mental states). It should be managed by treating the other problem, which is usually primary.

C. Hypertension in the obviously pregnant patient (> 20 weeks) should raise the question of preeclampsia and may need treatment with magnesium sulfate if associated with altered mental status or seizures.

D. Diastolic pressures and mean arterial pressures are much more important in determining danger of severe hypertension than is systolic pressure. These are poorly measured in the field. The diagnosis of "malignant" hypertension is not based on numerical levels, but rather on microscopic changes in blood vessels and damage to organs, which place this disease beyond the scope of prehospital care.

E. Don't forget that false elevation of BP can result from a cuff which is too small for the patient. The cuff should cover 1/3 to 1/2 of the upper arm and the bladder should completely encircle the arm.

F. Hypertension is seen in severe head injury and intracranial bleeding, and is thought to be a protective response which increases perfusion to the brain. Treatment should be directed at the intracranial process, not the blood pressure.

NEUROLOGIC DEFICIT

Specific information needed

A. Present history – when last well, where found, sequence of deficits, antecedent symptoms such as headache, head trauma, or seizure.

B. Past history – stroke, seizures, diabetes, cardiovascular disease, medications, drug or alcohol abuse.

Specific objective findings

A. Vital signs. Level of consciousness. Temperature.

B. Movement and symmetry of face, extremities.

C. Medical alert tags.

D. Signs of dehydration or of adrenaline effect (diaphoresis, tremor, tachycardia).

E. Signs of trauma.

Treatment

A. Ensure airway. Nasopharyngeal airway may be particularly useful.

B. Suction frequently and assist ventilations if needed.

C. O_2, moderate flow (4–6 L/min). Titrate to pulse oximetry > 90%.

D. IV – Saline lock or NS, TKO.

E. Monitor cardiac rhythm.

F. Consider hypoglycemia. If suggestive:

    1. Test blood for glucose level.

    2. Administer oral dextrose or bolus of dextrose 50%, 50 ml, IV in secure vein, if glucose level < 60 mg/dl.

G. Transport in lateral recumbent position to protect airway.

H. Monitor vitals during transport.

Specific precautions

A. Not all neurologic deficits are caused by stroke. Look for treatable medical conditions – hypoglycemia, hypothermia, hypoxia, and hyperthermia. Hypotension with resultant poor cerebral blood flow may be another reversible cause of neurologic deficit. Fluid administration or PASG inflation in the elderly can be risky, however. Consult base physician.

B. Hypoglycemia is the great mimic. It can present with: seizures, coma, behavior problems, intoxication, confusion or stroke-like picture with focal deficits (particularly in elderly patients).

C. A patient with a stroke can present with aphasia (inability to talk) and still be completely alert. Talk to the patient, explain everything that you are doing, and avoid comments that you would not want to hear yourself.

POISONS AND OVERDOSES

Specific information needed

A. Is there any potential exposure risk to rescuers?

B. Type of ingestion – What, when, and how much was ingested? Bring the poison, the container, sample of emesis, all medications and everything questionable in the area with the patient to the emergency department.

C. Reason for ingestion – think of child neglect, attempted suicide.

D. Symptoms – nausea, burning, eye irritation, respiratory distress, sleepiness.

E. Past history – medications, diseases.

F. Action taken by bystanders – induced emesis? "Antidote" given?

Specific objective findings

A. Vital signs.

B. Airway – clear, open, and judge adequacy of ventilations.

C. Level of consciousness and neurologic status – check frequently.

D. Breath odor, increased salivation, oral burns.

E. Skin – sweating, evidence of skin burns.

F. Eye irritation.

G. Systemic signs – vomitus, dysrhythmias, lung findings.

Treatment

A. External contamination

   1. Protect rescuer from contamination. Wear appropriate gloves and clothing. Contact Hazardous Materials Unit with any indication of persistent risk.

   2. Remove all clothing and any solid chemical which might provide continuing contamination.

   3. Assess and treat for associated injuries if possible.

   4. Decontaminate patient using running water for 15 minutes prior to transport.

5. Wrap burned area in clean, dry cloth for transport after irrigation. Keep patient as warm as possible after decontamination.

6. Check eyes particularly for exposure and rinse with free-flowing water for 15 minutes.

7. Evaluate for systemic symptoms which might be caused by chemical contamination. Contact base for possible treatment.

8. Remove rings, bracelets, constricting bands.

9. Consult base or Poison Control Center (PCC) for special treatment or procedures if needed.

B. Internal ingestion

1. *If transport time > 20 minutes, contact base to consider administering charcoal or ipecac orally if no contraindications exist. *(Do not administer both)*.

   Charcoal Dose: 1 gm/kg orally in adult, 1 gm/kg orally in children.

   Ipecac Dose: 30 ml orally in adult, 15 ml orally in child over one year.

   Contraindications include unconscious, or poorly responsive patient, no gag reflex, or ingested caustics or hydrocarbons.

2. If patient is poorly responsive or has depressed respirations:

   a. Assess and support ABCs.

   b. O_2, high flow (10–15 L/min). Titrate to pulse oximetry > 90% if possible.

   c. Support patient on side and protect airway.

   d. IV – volume expander (NS or RL), TKO.

   e. Test blood for glucose level. Administer dextrose 50%, 50 ml, IV in secure vein, if glucose level < 60 mg/dl.

   f. Naloxone, 2 mg IV in adult for suspected narcotic toxicity.

   g. Monitor cardiac rhythm if antidepressant or cardiac drugs ingested.

    h. *Consider sodium bicarbonate if: widened QRS, prolonged P-R, or ventricular dysrhythmias on monitor after tricyclic antidepressant OD.

  3. Monitor vitals and level of consciousness during transport. Do not leave patient unattended.

Specific precautions

A. There are few specific "antidotes". Product labels and home kits can be misleading and dangerous. Watch the ABCs, *these* are important.

B. Do not neutralize acids with alkalis. Do not neutralize alkalis with acids. These "treatments" cause heat-releasing chemical reactions which can further injure the GI track.

C. A commonly missed external contamination is gasoline. Be sure that gasoline spilled on trauma victims is washed off promptly and clothing removed to prevent irritant burns.

D. Inhalation poisoning is particularly dangerous to rescuers. Recognize an environment with continuing contamination and extricate rapidly or avoid altogether.

Telephone Number of Local Poison Control Center

RESPIRATORY DISTRESS

Specific information needed

A. History – acute change or injury, slow deterioration.

B. Past history – chronic lung or heart problems or known diagnosis, medications, home oxygen, past allergic reactions, recent surgery, diabetes.

C. Associated symptoms – chest pain, cough, hand or mouth paresthesias, fever.

Specific objective findings

A. Vital signs.

B. Oxygenation – color, level of consciousness.

C. Ventilatory effort – accessory muscle use, forward position, pursed lips.

D. Neurologic signs – slurred speech, impaired consciousness, evidence of drug/alcohol ingestion.

E. Signs of upper airway obstruction – hoarseness, drooling, exaggerated chest wall movements, inspiratory stridor.

F. Signs of congestive failure – neck vein distention in upright position, wet crackling lung sounds, peripheral edema.

G. Breath sounds – clear, decreased, wet or crackling (rales), wheezing, or rhonchi.

H. Hives, upper airway edema.

I. Evidence of trauma – crepitus of neck or chest, bruising, steering wheel damage, penetrating wounds.

Treatment

A. Put patient in position of comfort (usually upright).

B. O_2 – flow as necessary for patient comfort. Administer high flow oxygen for respiratory distress with no evidence COPD. Titrate to pulse oximetry > 90% if possible.

In COPD use O_2, 1–2 L/min or 1 L/min over home flow. Increase by 1–2 L/min as needed if cyanosis persists. Titrate to comfort, be prepared to assist ventilations if necessary.

C. Assess and consider treatment for the following problems if respiratory distress is severe and patient does not respond to proper positioning and administration of O_2:

1. *Asthma:*

    a. IV – volume expander (NS or RL), TKO if respiratory distress severe.

    b. Monitor cardiac rhythm in patients over 40.

    c. Albuterol, 2.5 mg by nebulizer (repeat as needed).

    d. *Consider epinephrine 1:1,000 SQ, 0.3 ml in adult who does not respond to repeated albuterol.

2. *Pulmonary edema:*

    a. Sit patient up, legs dangling if possible.

    b. IV – Saline lock or D5W, TKO.

    c. Monitor cardiac rhythm.

    d. Nitroglycerin, 0.4 mg, SL. (Repeat every 3 minutes as long as systolic BP > 90.)

    e. Contact base to consider:

        1. *Furosemide, 20–40 mg IV.

        2. *Morphine sulfate, 2–4 mg IV; may repeat every 3 minutes, not to exceed 0.2 mg/kg.

    f. Assist ventilations and consider intubation if patient has altered mentation.

3. *Chronic lung disease* with deterioration:

    a. O_2, low flow (1–2 L/min or 1 L/min > home flow).

    b. Monitor cardiac rhythm.

    c. IV – Saline lock or D5W, TKO.

    d. Albuterol, 2.5 mg by nebulizer (repeat as needed).

4. *Pneumothorax:* watch for signs of tension. If patient deteriorating rapidly, consider decompression.

D. If diagnosis is unclear, place patient in position of comfort, and administer oxygen. Transport rapidly for severe distress.

E. Prepare to assist ventilations if patient fatigues or develops altered mentation, or if respiratory arrest occurs.

Specific precautions

A. Don't over diagnose "hyperventilation" in the field. Your patient could have a pulmonary embolus or other serious problem. Give them the benefit of the doubt. Treatment with oxygen will not harm the patient with hyperventilation, and it will keep you from underestimating the problem.

B. Wheezing in older persons may be due to pulmonary edema ("Cardiac Asthma"). Consider also pulmonary embolus, or foreign body as less common causes of wheezing.

C. Do not overtreat the COPD patient with oxygen. Diminished anxiety and respiratory struggle may presage a full cardiopulmonary arrest. Start with 1–2 L/min (or 1 L/min over home O_2 flow). O_2 may be increased in 1–2 L/min increments if cyanosis or air hunger still present.

D. Patients with COPD and respiratory distress are commonly seen in the field and are difficult to evaluate. Pulmonary edema is rare, and treatment in the field with morphine and furosemide is contraindicated in persons with evidence of COPD. Acute problems may be due to bronchospasm, but epinephrine may have undesirable side effects. Pneumothorax may occur but is difficult to diagnose. Albuterol is relatively safe in these patients and can be administered as a constant (or repetitive) nebulization. Occasionally the patient with COPD must be transported rapidly with supportive care only. You cannot clear acute-superimposed-upon-chronic respiratory failure in a few minutes. Intubate only for respiratory arrest. Discuss the patient with base physician if specific modes of treatment seem appropriate.

TABLE 2-5. BREATH SOUNDS IN RESPIRATORY DISTRESS

Auscultation	Location	Possible diagnosis
Clear	Bilateral	MI, metabolic, pulmonary embolus, anxiety, toxin.
Decreased	Bilateral	COPD
	Localized	COPD, pneumothorax, pulmonary embolus, pneumonia.
Crackles (rales) (inspiration)	Bilateral	Pulmonary edema, pneumonia.
	Localized	Pneumonia, pulmonary edema.
Wheezes (expiration)	Bilateral	Asthma, occasionally pulmonary edema, embolus.
	Localized	Foreign body, embolus, COPD.
Rhonchi (coarse, wet sounds)	Bilateral	Bronchitis, COPD.

SEIZURES

Specific information needed
A. Seizure history – onset, time interval, previous seizures, type of seizure.

B. Medical history – especially head trauma, diabetes, headaches, drugs, alcohol, medications, pregnancy.

Specific objective findings
A. Vital signs.

B. Description of seizure activity.

C. Level of consciousness.

D. Head and mouth trauma.

E. Incontinence.

F. Air temperature, patient temperature.

G. Skin color and moisture.

Treatment
A. Airway – ensure patency – nasopharyngeal airways useful. Note: Do not *force* anything between the teeth. Do not use esophageal obturator airway.

B. O_2, moderate flow (4–6 L/min). Titrate to pulse oximetry > 90%.

C. Suction as needed.

D. If seizure persists or patient not alert:

   1. Protect patient from injury.

   2. Check pulse immediately after seizure stops. Keep patient on side.

   3. IV – Saline lock, NS, or RL, TKO.

   4. Test blood for glucose level.

   5. Administer dextrose 50%, 50 ml IV into secure vein, if glucose level < 60 mg/dl.

   6. Administer naloxone, 2 mg IV for suspected narcotic toxicity.

   7. *Consider diazepam, 5–10 mg (not to exceed 0.3 mg/kg) *slowly* IV, for status seizure activity.

8. *Consider magnesium sulfate 1–2 gm slowly IV for the pregnant patient with suspected eclampsia.

E. Monitor cardiac rhythm.

F. Keep in lateral recumbent position for transport.

G. Monitor vitals.

Specific precautions

A. Move hazardous materials away from patient. Restrain patient only if needed to prevent injury. Protect patient's head.

B. Trauma to tongue is unlikely to cause serious problems. Trauma to teeth *may*. Attempts to force an airway into the patient's mouth can completely obstruct airway. Do not use bite sticks.

C. Seizure can be due to lack of glucose or oxygen to the brain, as well as to the irritable focus we associate with epilepsy. Hypoxia from transient dysrhythmia or cardiac arrest (particularly in younger patients) may cause seizure and should be treated promptly. Don't forget to check for pulse once a seizure terminates.

D. Hypoxic seizures can also be caused by simple faint, either when the tongue obstructs the airway in the supine position, or when overly helpful bystanders "prop" the patient upright or elevate the head prematurely.

E. Alcohol-related seizures are common, but cannot be differentiated from other causes of seizure in the field. Assessment in the intoxicated patient should still include consideration of hypoglycemia and all other potential causes.

F. In patients over the age of 50, seizures may be due to dysrhythmias or stroke. Of these, dysrhythmia is the most important to recognize in the field.

G. Medical personnel are often called to assist epileptics who seize in public. If the patient clears completely, is taking his medications, has his own physician, and is experiencing his usual frequency of seizures, transport may be unnecessary. Consult your base physician.

H. Seizures in pregnant patients (or even those who are recently delivered) may be the presenting sign of eclampsia or toxemia of pregnancy. Seizures in pregnant patients are better treated by administration of magnesium sulfate.

SHOCK: MEDICAL

Specific information needed

A. Onset – gradual or sudden, precipitating cause or event.

B. Associated symptoms – itching, peripheral or facial edema, thirst, weakness, respiratory distress, abdominal or chest pain, dizziness on standing.

C. History – allergies, medications, bloody vomitus or stools, significant medical diseases, history of recent trauma, last menstrual period, vaginal bleeding, fever.

Specific objective findings

A. Vital signs – pulse > 120 (occasionally < 50); BP < 90 systolic.

B. Mental status – sleepy, apathy, confusion, restlessness, mania.

C. Skin – flushed, pale, sweaty, cool or warm, hives, or other rash.

D. Signs of trauma, particularly blunt.

E. Signs of pump failure (back-up pressure) – jugular venous distention in upright position, wet lung sounds, peripheral edema (indicates chronic pump failure).

Treatment

A. Stop exsanguinating hemorrhage.

B. Apply PASG to stretcher before loading patient.

C. O_2, high flow (10–15 L/min). Titrate to pulse oximetry > 90% if possible.

D. Cover patient to avoid excess heat loss. Do not overbundle.

E. Assess for hypovolemia. Treat as indicated.

    1. IV – volume expander (NS or RL), large bore, TKO or as directed.

    2. Consider PASG inflation or fluid challenge.

F. Assess for cardiogenic cause (see Table 2.6):

    1. If P > 150, treat tachydysrhythmia according to protocol.

    2. If P < 60, treat bradydysrhythmia according to protocol.

    3. If distended neck veins, chest pain, or other evidence of cardiac cause:

    a. Position of comfort.

    b. Be prepared to assist ventilations or initiate CPR.

    c. IV – volume expander (NS or RL), large bore, TKO or as directed.

    d. Monitor cardiac rhythm.

    e. *Consider tension pneumothorax. Treat as appropriate.

    f. *Consider dopamine drip – begin at 5 mcg/kg/min IV.

    g. *Contact base to consider PASG inflation, fluid challenge, or other treatment.

    h. Transport rapidly for definitive diagnosis and treatment.

G. Consider anaphylaxis. Treat as appropriate.

H. If no evidence of specific cause, institute general treatment measures:

    1. Place patient supine, elevate legs 10–12 inches. (If respiratory distress results, leave patient in position of comfort.)

    2. Inflate PASG according to protocol if BP < 90.

    3. IV – volume expander (NS or RL), large bore, 20 ml/kg rapid IV, then TKO or as directed.

I. Monitor VS, cardiac rhythm, and level of consciousness during transport.

Specific precautions

A. Shock in a cardiac patient may still represent hypovolemia. Administer small fluid boluses (250 ml) and monitor response closely. Watch for signs/symptoms of pulmonary edema.

B. Mixed forms of shock (see Table 2-6) are treated as hypovolemia, but the other factors contributing to the low perfusion should be considered. Neurogenic shock is caused by relative hypovolemia as blood vessels lose tone, either from cord trauma, drug overdose, or sepsis. Cardiac depressant factors can also be involved. Some treatments are quite controversial, including steroids and naloxone in high doses. Anaphylaxis is a mixed form of shock with hypovolemic, neurogenic, and cardiac depressant components. Epinephrine is used in addition to fluid load.

SYNCOPE

Specific information needed

A. History of the event – precipitating factors, onset, duration, seizure activity. Was the patient sitting, standing, or lying? Pregnant?

B. Past history – medications, diseases, prior syncope, trauma.

C. Associated symptoms – dizziness, nausea, chest or back pain, abdominal pain, headache, palpitations.

Specific objective findings

A. Vital signs.

B. Neurologic status – level of consciousness, residual neurologic deficit.

C. Signs of head trauma, mouth trauma, incontinence.

D. Neck stiffness.

Treatment

A. Position of comfort. *Do not* sit patient up prematurely. Supine or lateral positioning if not completely alert.

B. Monitor vital signs and level of consciousness closely for changes or recurrence.

C. Consider hypoglycemia. If suggestive:

    1. Test blood for glucose level.

    2. Administer oral dextrose or bolus of dextrose 50%, 50 ml, IV in secure vein if glucose level < 60 mg/dl.

D. If vital signs unstable or symptoms persist:

    1. O_2, high flow (10–15 L/min). Titrate to pulse oximetry > 90% if possible.

    2. Keep patient supine, elevate legs 10–12 inches.

    3. Apply PASG and inflate if signs of hypovolemia and systolic BP < 90.

    4. IV – volume expander (NS or RL), TKO or as directed.

    5. Monitor cardiac rhythm.

TABLE 2-6. CAUSES OF MEDICAL SHOCK

Mechanism Causes	Differential Symptoms
Hypovolemia	
Dehydration	
Vomiting, diarrhea	suggestive illness
Diabetes with hyperglycemia thirst;	diabetes, illness,increased urine or fever
Blood loss	female, 12–50 years,
Ectopic pregnancy	abdominal pain, missed period
GI bleed	bloody vomitus,black or red stool.
Abdominal aneurysm	severe back or abdominal pain, syncope.
Vaginal bleeding	suggestive history, miscarriage, or abortion.
Intra-abdominal bleeding	trauma – abdomen, back or shoulder pain
Cardiogenic	
Dysrhythmia	palpitations
Pericardial tamponade	chest cancer, blunt or penetrating trauma
Tension pneumothorax	respiratory distress, COPD, trauma
Myocardial failure	chest pain, history of congestive heart failure
Pulmonary embolus	sudden respiratory distress, chest pain
Mixed	
Sepsis	fever, elderly, urinary symptoms or catheter
Drug overdose	suggestive history
Anaphylaxis	itching, mouth swelling, dizziness, exposure to allergen, rash, respiratory distress

TABLE 2-6. Continued

Differential Findings	Specific Advanced Treatment
poor skin turgor, sunken eyes dry mucus membranes, vomiting, diarrhea	IV fluid bolus, 20 ml/kg,
signs of dehydration as above, fever, medical alert tag	NS or RL
abdominal pain, hypotension pallor, vasoconstrictio	1. PASG inflation per protocol, if indicated
red or black vomitus or stool, hypotension or tachycardia, pallor, vasoconstriction abdominal distention, pulsatile mass	2. IV fluid bolus, 20 ml/kg, NS or RL
heavy vaginal bleeding	
abdominal tenderness, rigidity, pallor	
pulse < 60 or > 150	Treat rhythm
jugular vein distention, distant heart sounds, narrow pulse pressure	Cautious IV fluid bolus, 10 ml/kg
hyperinflated chest, decreased breath sounds, severe respiratory distress	Rapid transport Needle decompression
neck veins flat or distended, pulmonary edema	Dopamine drip
dyspnea, wheezing or decreased breath sounds	Rapid transport CPR if needed
fever, vasodilatation	IV fluid bolus, 10 ml/kg
depressed respirations, lack of vasoconstriction suicide evidence	IV fluid bolus, 10 ml/kg naloxone 2 mg IV
hives, wheezing, flushed, sudden collapse	IV fluid bolus, 20 ml/kg Epinephrine, 1 ml 1:10,000 (adult) IV

Specific precautions

A. Syncope is by definition a transient state of unconsciousness from which the patient has recovered. If the patient is still unconscious, treat as coma. If the patient is confused, treat according to Altered Mental State Protocol.

B. Most syncope is vasovagal, with dizziness progressing to faint over several minutes. Recumbent position should be sufficient to restore vital signs and level of consciousness to normal.

C. Syncope which occurs without warning or while in a recumbent position is potentially serious, and often caused by dysrhythmia.

D. Patients over the age of 40 with syncope, even though apparently normal, should be transported. In middle-aged or elderly patients, syncope can be due to a number of potentially serious problems. The most important to monitor and recognize are: dysrhythmias, occult GI bleeding, seizure, or leaking abdominal aortic aneurysm.

VAGINAL BLEEDING

Specific information needed
A. Symptoms – cramping, passage of clots or tissue, dizziness, weakness, thirst.

B. Present history – duration, amount, last menstrual period (normal or abnormal), birth control method. If pregnant – due date. If postpartum – time and place of delivery, current medications.

C. Past history – medications, bleeding problems, pregnancies, allergies, sexual assault.

Specific objective findings
A. Vital signs.

B. Evidence of blood clots, or tissue fragments (bring tissue to ED).

C. Signs of hypovolemic shock – altered mental status, hypotension, tachycardia, sweating, skin pallor.

D. Fever.

Treatment
A. O_2, moderate flow (4–6 L/min). Titrate to pulse oximetry > 90%.

B. If BP < 90 systolic and signs of hypovolemic shock:

    1. With early or no apparent pregnancy:

        a. Elevate legs 10 inches and keep patient warm.

        b. IV – volume expander (NS or RL), large bore, wide open 20 ml/kg, further fluids as directed.

    2. With mid or late pregnancy:

        a. Position left lateral recumbent and keep patient warm.

        b. IV en route – volume expander (NS or RL), large bore, wide open 20 ml/kg, further fluids as directed.

        c. Transport rapidly if bleeding severe.

    3. If patient postpartum (within 24 hours):

        a. Massage uterus.

    b. IV – as above for hypovolemic shock.

    c. *Consider oxytocin administration.

C. If BP > 90 systolic and patient stable, transport non-emergent.

D. Monitor vital signs during transport.

Specific precautions

A. Amount of vaginal bleeding is difficult to estimate. Visual estimates from sheets or towels can be misleading. Try to get an estimate of number of saturated menstrual pads in previous 6 hours. Discreet inspection of the perineum may be useful to determine if clots or tissue are being passed. *Vaginal exam in the field is not indicated.*

B. A patient in shock from vaginal bleeding should be treated like any patient with hypovolemic shock. Vaginal bleeding in late pregnancy, however, may make consideration of appropriate destination more pertinent. Any complication of pregnancy should be transported to the nearest facility that can appropriately manage those complications.

C. If patient could be pregnant, bring in any tissue which has been passed. Laboratory analysis may be important in determining status of pregnancy.

D. Consider possibility of sexual assault in the very young or infirm.

E. Always consider pregnancy as a cause of vaginal bleeding. The history may contain inaccuracies, denial, or wishful thinking. The only patients who "can't be pregnant" are male.

VOMITING OR DIARRHEA

Specific information needed
A. Frequency, duration of vomiting, diarrhea.

B. Presence of blood in vomitus, stool.

C. Associated symptoms – abdominal pain, weakness, confusion.

D. Medication ingestion.

E. Past medical history – diabetes, cardiac disease, abdominal problems, alcoholism, recent travel, several persons affected.

Specific objective findings
A. Vital signs.

B. Color of vomitus, diarrhea, presence of blood.

C. Abdomen – tenderness, guarding, rigidity, distention.

D. Signs of dehydration – poor skin turgor, tearless eyes, dry mucous membranes, confusion.

Treatment
A. Position patient: left lateral recumbent if vomiting; otherwise supine. Protect airway as needed.

B. O_2, moderate flow (4–6 L/min). Titrate to pulse oximetry > 90%.

C. Nothing by mouth.

D. If BP > 90 systolic, *consider droperidol 0.025 mg/kg slowly IV for intractable vomiting.

E. If BP < 90 systolic and signs of hypovolemic shock:

   1. Elevate legs 10–12 inches.

   2. IV – volume expander (NS or RL), large bore, 20 ml/kg wide open, further fluids as directed.

F. Monitor vital signs during transport.

Specific precautions
A. Vomiting or diarrhea may be symptoms of a more serious problem, but all cause some degree of hypovolemia. The most serious causes are GI bleed or other intra-abdominal catastrophe.

A rare cardiac patient may also present with vomiting or diarrhea as the predominant symptom.

B. Be sure to use an adequate emesis basin. Support the patient's head when he is vomiting.

C. Vomiting as an isolated symptom should always be suspected to be secondary. Consider ingestion, cardiac disease or other serious conditions. May be the initial presentation of CO poisoning.

D. The vast majority of persons with vomiting and diarrhea have become sick over days, not minutes. Unless severely ill, they do not require lights-and-siren transport or advanced field treatment.

E. Dehydration may be particularly severe in children with simple vomiting and diarrhea. IVs may be very difficult to start, particularly with infants. Transport for definitive treatment is usually best.

F. Blood in the GI tract is an irritant. It causes vomiting and diarrhea. Only if upper tract bleeding is extremely brisk will the blood reach the rectum undigested (i.e., still bright red). GI bleeders may be very sick and hypovolemic without showing an obvious source of their problem.

3

PEDIATRIC TREATMENT PROTOCOLS

PEDIATRIC TREATMENT OVERVIEW

Pediatric patients are not just "small people". They have unique needs and problems that will affect prehospital as well as hospital care. These differences are all the more important to remember, because infants and children make up a small part of our patient population and opportunities to practice assessment and management skills are infrequent. In addition, the pediatric emergency is rarely preceded by chronic disease. If intervention is swift and effective, the child can often be restored to full health. This makes the psychological burden and reward for us as providers all the greater.

The following principles should be remembered:

A. Airways are smaller, softer, and easier to obstruct or collapse.

B. Respiratory reserve is small. Minor insults such as improper positioning, vomitus, stomach filled with air, or airway narrowing can lead to major problems.

C. Circulatory reserve is also small. The loss of one unit of blood is sufficient to account for severe shock or death in an infant. Conversely, 500 ml of unnecessary fluid can result in acute pulmonary edema.

D. Vital signs and level of consciousness are difficult to assess. History, a high index of suspicion, and "soft signs" can be critical. Listen to the parents. They know when changes have occurred, even if they have difficulty expressing what has changed.

E. Nutritional reserves are limited, particularly in younger infants. Dextrose should be added to infant IVs when possible. D5RL or D5NS can be carried as premixed IV solutions, or made by adding 50 ml of 50% dextrose to 500 ml NS or RL.

F. Electrolyte solutions should always be used in pediatric IVs. D5W is *not* indicated for infants or children.

G. The proper size of equipment is very important because of the child's poor cardiorespiratory reserve. A complete selection of laryngoscope blades, ET tubes, suction catheters and IV catheters is essential for optimal care.

H. Pediatric equipment and drugs should be stored separately so they can be found easily when needed.

I. Pediatric resuscitation skills must be practiced to be ready when needed. In addition, protocols should be kept simple and procedures with poor likelihood of success should be left to the hospital setting *if* simpler support and rapid transport will suffice to maintain the patient.

INFANT AND CHILD RESUSCITATION

Specific information needed
A. History – what happened, when was child found, recent illness.

B. Past history – diseases, medications.

C. Surroundings – evidence of abuse, neglect, poisoning.

Specific objective findings
A. Absence of consciousness.

B. Terminal or no respirations.

C. Absence of central pulse (carotid or femoral).

D. Color, temperature.

E. Signs of trauma.

Treatment
A. Open airway and attempt ventilation.

B. If airway obstructed:

    1. Attempt to visualize airway with laryngoscope and remove any obvious foreign body.

    2. Reposition airway.

    3. Attempt to ventilate.

    4. If unsuccessful, administer up to 5 subdiaphragmatic abdominal thrusts (child) or up to 5 back blows and 5 chest thrusts (infant).

    5. Remove apparent foreign body, or

    6. Repeat steps 1–5 if needed.

    7. Consider needle cricothyrotomy if obstruction unrelieved.

C. Check pulse once ventilations established. Begin chest compressions if no pulse.

D. Check rhythm with monitor or quick-look paddles.

VENTRICULAR FIBRILLATION

1. Defibrillate with 2 joules/kg, pediatric paddles.

2. If no response to initial shock repeat immediately with 4 joules/kg.

3. If no response, shock again with 4 joules/kg.

4. If no response, intubate and hyperventilate at 30 breaths/min.

5. If no response, administer:

   Epinephrine (1:10,000), 0.1 ml/kg IV or (1:1,000) 0.1 ml/kg via ET, (ET dose is 10 times IV dose).

   Lidocaine 1 mg/kg IV or I0.

6. Assess for hypovolemia. If possible – start IV or IO, volume expander (RL or NS) administer 20 ml/kg.

BRADYCARDIA OR SLOW PEA

1. Oxygenate and hyperventilate. Intubate.

2. Compress chest if heart rate is < 80/minute in infant or < 60/minute in child.

3. IV or IO – volume expander (RL or NS).

4. Treat for possible hypovolemia. Start IV or IO – volume expander (RL or NS), administer 20 ml/kg rapidly.

5. Consider:

   a. Epinephrine (1:10,000) 0.1 ml/kg IV or 0.1 ml/kg (1:1,000) via ET.

   b. Atropine, 0.02 mg/kg IV or ET.

   c. *Sodium bicarbonate 1 mEq/kg IV.

ASYSTOLE

1. Oxygenate and hyperventilate. Intubate.

2. IV – volume expander (RL or NS).

3. Treat for possible hypovolemia. Start IV – volume expander (RL or NS), administer 20 ml/kg rapidly.

4. Consider:

    a. Epinephrine (1:10,000) 0.1 ml/kg IV or (1:1,000) 0.1 ml/kg ET. May repeat IV Epinephrine 0.1 – 0.2 ml/kg (1:10,000) in 3–5 minutes.

    b. *Sodium bicarbonate 1 mEq/kg IV.

E. Transport rapidly for further resuscitation with CPR in progress.

Specific precautions

A. Pediatric arrests are most likely to be primary respiratory events. The rescuer's primary attention, therefore, must be directed to ensure both airway and good ventilations before any concerns for the cardiac rhythm. *Any* cardiac rhythm can spontaneously convert to NSR in a well-ventilated child.

B. Infants and children have a much greater capacity than adults to recover from cardiorespiratory arrest. CPR should be started if there is any possibility of recovery. If the chances appear poor, basic CPR with rapid transport will still allow the relatives to receive the emotional and social support of the hospital environment. Conversely, children who are cold, rigid and mottled should be left at the scene after notification and arrival of responsible law enforcement personnel.

C. SIDS (Sudden Infant Death Syndrome) will be one of the most frequent causes of cardiorespiratory arrest in infants between the ages of 1 month to 1 year. The parents or caretakers will have a great deal of guilt feelings. If these feelings are recognized and addressed it can help prevent some of the long-term effects of this devastating occurrence. Unfortunately, SIDS can be very hard to distinguish from child abuse and vice versa. Therefore it is most important not to be judgmental or suggest a diagnosis when there is not enough information to be accurate.

D. Cardiorespiratory arrest in a trauma situation (as with an adult) is best treated with rapid transport with CPR en route. IVs may be established and fluids administered during transport.

E. The most successful infant resuscitations occur *before* a full cardiopulmonary arrest. Assess infants carefully and assist with airway, breathing, and circulatory problems *before* the arrest occurs to improve the overall care to the pediatric patient.

F. The current recommendations from the American Heart Association (AHA 10/92) for obstructed airway are for abdominal thrusts in children over the age of one year only. Infants less than one year should be treated with both back blows and chest thrusts. The Pediatric Advanced Life Support (PALS) course is recommended for learning technique. However, paramedics or advanced EMTs should not feel restricted, but should use the laryngoscope early in an attempt to visualize the foreign body.

G. Note the following differences in pediatric drug doses:

Sodium bicarbonate is administered as half-strength solution (4.2%) for infants less than 10 kg. Use premixed pediatric ampules or dilute adult strength 1:1 with saline. Dose is 1 mEq/kg or 2 ml/kg of the 4.2% solution.

Epinephrine is given in the 1:10,000 strength IV or the 1:1,000 strength for ET administration.

Dextrose 25% (dilute 1:1 with saline or sterile water), 2–4 ml/kg of 25% solution.

For IVs – RL or NS is preferred.

H. The Broselow Pediatric Resuscitation Tape is a relatively new, simple and effective way to have multiple bits of data available to assist with infant and pediatric resuscitation. The tape is designed to place beside the youngster. Drugs and equipment are pre measured and calculated such that by reading off the tape at the appropriate length of the patient, the approximate weight is given with equipment size listing and critical drug dosages. Its use is recommended.

NEONATAL RESUSCITATION

Specific information needed

A. History of mother – age, due date, prenatal care, previous pregnancies and problems, medications, duration of labor, foul-smelling or stained amniotic fluid.

B. History of infant – if already delivered, when was delivery. How has infant behaved since delivery. What has been done for infant.

Specific objective findings

A. Vital signs, APGAR score at 1, 5 and 10 minutes.

B. Temperature or warmth of skin. Color. Spontaneous movement.

C. Meconium (brown/green/black stool fragments) in amniotic fluid or in newborn's airway.

Treatment

A. If baby is not delivered and head is not appearing at vaginal opening with contractions, transport rapidly and prepare to stop for delivery en route if situation changes.

B. If baby is not delivered, but head visible with contractions (crowning), delivery is imminent.

    1. Set up clean or sterile area for delivering baby:

        a. Place sterile or clean drape between mother's legs.

        b. Set sterile clamps, scissors, and suction on drape.

        c. Put on sterile gloves.

        d. Assign one attendant to mother, second to infant.

    2. As infant's head is delivering, put very gentle pressure against it with several fingers flat against head (not finger tips) to prevent an explosive delivery.

    3. As soon as head has delivered, use bulb suction to clear mouth (Figure 2-1, p. 45) (to back of mouth only, not throat) then nose (before delivery of infant's body if possible).

    4. Suction immediately after delivery also, using bulb syringe to suction first the mouth, then the nose. Administer O_2 near face and stimulate by drying with clean towel or blanket.

    5. If apparent meconium – suction airway under direct

    laryngoscopic vision using catheter or ET tube to remove all visible meconium from the airway.

C. After baby delivered, assess general appearance.

  1. *If infant pink, with good cry and active movement* (APGAR 8–10):

    a. Wrap in clean, dry blanket.

    b. Keep infant level with perineum.

    c. Clamp cord in two places 8–10 inches from infant.

    d. Cut cord between clamps.

    e. Bundle infant with mother, continue to monitor.

  2. *If infant color poor, weak cry, or limp* (APGAR 7 or less):

    a. Hold O_2 tubing near infant's face.

    b. Keep infant warm.

    c. Continue to stimulate with suction and drying.

    d. Assist ventilation with bag-valve-mask using 100% O_2 by positive pressure if respirations are inadequate, heart rate is < 100, or central cyanosis persists despite 100% oxygen. Assist at a rate of 40 to 60 breaths/min.

    e. Suction trachea under direct vision if any meconium remains in airway. Intubate if respirations poor.

    f. CPR if heart rate < 60/minute and unresponsive to ventilations.

    g. Clamp cord when infant level with perineum.

    h. Transport as soon as possible with Porta Warmer or other infant warming system.

Specific precautions

A. Neonatal resuscitation, unlike most other resuscitation situations, requires careful attention to temperature. For neonates the management priorities are:

  A Airway

  B Breathing

  C Circulation

  T Temperature

The newborn has very poor temperature control and circulatory and respiratory status are often entirely dependent on core temperature. If infant requires resuscitation, place in dry blanket on Porta-Warmer or other infant warming system. Wrap warmer and infant with silver swaddling if possible to aid in heat conservation.

B. Avoid overstimulation of the back of the pharynx during suctioning. This may cause bradycardia in newborn. Do suction nares, as babies breathe only through nose for the first few months.

C. If thick meconium is present in upper airway or an adequate airway cannot be obtained, use laryngoscope and suction through the endotracheal tube to clear airway under direct vision and avoid contamination of the lungs with meconium as much as possible. This should only be done under dire circumstances, since it is time-consuming and can cause heat loss and hypoxia – minimize the time of suctioning.

D. Airway management should be kept as simple as possible. Oxygen delivered by tube to the area of baby's face is usually all that is needed to aid in resuscitation. Bag-valve-mask respirations and endotracheal intubation should be considered only if initial oxygen provision fails to revive the neonate.

E. Infants, particularly preemies, are very fragile. In most instances, basic stabilization by airway control, suctioning, temperature conservation and CPR en route to the hospital is recommended. This is not the time to try IVs, drugs, or other ALS procedures in the field.

F. The DeLee suction was previously recommended as it allowed good airway suction to occur with minimal equipment. However, recent guidelines from the American Heart Association (AHA) recommend against "techniques that involve mouth suction by the health care provider". The preferred method at present is a bulb syringe or 8–10 French suction catheter on *low* suction.

PEDIATRIC RESPIRATORY DISTRESS

Specific information needed
A. Present symptoms – sudden or gradual onset.

B. History of oral exposures – toys, food, chemicals, etc.

C. Associated symptoms – cough, fever, upper respiratory symptoms, runny nose, sore throat, drooling, hoarseness.

D. Past medical problems.

E. Current medications.

Specific objective findings
A. Mental status – alert, agitated, confused, somnolent.

B. Respiratory effort – upper airway sounds, chest wall movement, use of accessory muscles, retractions (depressions between ribs on inspiration).

C. Audible breathing noise – wheezes, cough, crowing.

D. Lungs by auscultation – wheezes, crackles (wet sounds), clear lung fields, decreased breath sounds.

E. Other findings – drooling, fever, skin color.

Treatment
A. Put patient in position of comfort (usually upright).

B. If respiratory arrest – attempt to ventilate. Watch neck position carefully and adjust for maximum chest rise.

C. If patient has airway obstruction from foreign body:

    1. Encourage coughing efforts with partial obstruction.

    2. If no air movement, visualize airway with laryngoscope and remove any obvious foreign body.

    3. Reposition the airway.

    4. Attempt to ventilate.

    5. If unsuccessful, administer up to 5 subdiaphragmatic abdominal thrusts for children or 5 back blows and 5 chest thrusts for infants.

6. Reposition the airway and attempt to ventilate.

7. If unsuccessful, consider percutaneous cricothyrotomy with 14 g. angiocath if qualified.

D. Apply O_2, high flow (10–15 L/min or volume sufficient to keep bag inflated) for significant respiratory distress. Titrate to pulse oximetry > 90% if possible.

E. If patient is ventilating inadequately:

1. Assist ventilations as needed with bag-valve-mask and high flow oxygen.

2. Consider intubation if less invasive means are inadequate.

F. Assist and consider treatment for the following problems if respiratory distress is severe and patient does not respond to proper positioning and administration of O_2:

1. Croup

    a. *Administer racemic epinephrine 0.3–0.5 ml (depending on age) with 2 ml saline via nebulizer.

    b. Prepare to assist ventilations if child fatigues and is unable to maintain adequate ventilations.

2. Epiglottitis

    a. Allow patient to remain upright.

    b. Assist with removal of secretions if needed.

    c. *For long transport with severe distress, administer racemic epinephrine by updraft nebulizer as above.

    d. Prepare to assist ventilations.

3. Asthma

    a. Administer albuterol 1.5–3.0 ml 0.083% soln (1.5 ml under age 2, 3.0 ml over age 2) via nebulizer.

    b. *Administer epinephrine, 0.01 ml/kg of 1:1,000 SQ if no improvement with albuterol.

G. If diagnosis is unclear, transport patient rapidly with supplemental O_2, and prepare to assist ventilations if child becomes fatigued or sustains respiratory arrest.

Specific precautions

A. Children with croup, epiglottitis or laryngeal edema usually have respiratory arrest due to exhaustion or spasm. They may still be ventilated with pocket mask or bag-valve-mask (BVM) technique. Don't attempt intubation unless these techniques fail.

B. Intubation of children in the field is infrequently performed, and therefore carries some risk. Do not attempt intubation if a simpler skill will manage the airway.

C. Bag-valve-mask in small children carries the risk of excessive pressures and possible pneumothorax. It is easy to get overly excited and overventilate.

D. In respiratory distress of sudden onset, think of foreign body aspiration. The mouth is a major sensory organ for children (as well as others) and admits a multitude of obstructive hazards.

E. There may be a call to attend a child who has allegedly aspirated something that was in his or her mouth, but is now asymptomatic. This child may not need emergency intervention, but should be seen by a physician. Once the object has settled in the lung and is not irritating a major airway, it can rapidly become asymptomatic while still requiring removal to prevent further complications.

PEDIATRIC SEIZURES

Specific information needed
A. History – onset, duration of seizure, description of seizure activity, fever, recent illness.

B. Past history – immunizations, medications, previous seizures, diseases.

Specific objective findings
A. Vital signs.

B. Level of consciousness.

C. Fever, skin warmth, rash.

D. Signs of trauma.

Treatment
A. Ensure airway, suction as needed.

B. O_2, moderate flow (4–6 L/min). Titrate to pulse oximetry > 90%.

C. Remove excess clothing if patient feels febrile.

D. Keep patient on side. Protect from injury during confusion or further seizure activity.

E. If seizure persists or patient not alert:

1. IV – RL or NS. Start en route at TKO.

2. Test blood for glucose level.

3. If glucose level < 60 mg/dl, administer 2–4 ml/kg 25% dextrose into secure vein.

4. *Administer diazepam *slowly* IV 0.2 mg/kg (Max of 8 mg) if seizure activity persists. Diazepam may need to be administered rectally if IV access not available. *Be prepared to intubate if respiratory depression significant.*

F. Monitor vitals carefully en route. Keep patient on side.

Specific precautions
A. If patient is obviously febrile, you may use cool, wet towels during transport. *Do not delay transport for cooling.* Unbundling is often sufficient.

B. Unlike the adult with a diagnosis of epilepsy, a child who has had a seizure, even though alert on arrival of the paramedics, usually requires medical attention. He is best transported by ambulance. Do not be falsely reassured by return of normalcy. This is *not* true of the patient who has a history of seizures and is under the care of a physician for those seizures. Those patients can often be managed at home. The question must be asked, however, why emergency care was called for. Was this an unusual seizure? Or was this just an inexperienced (new) caretaker?

C. Seizures in children may not be the usual grand mal type. A staring, peculiar eye movement, unresponsiveness, or arm twitching may be the only clue. The parents are usually very sensitive to the abnormality and potential seriousness of the situation. Do not downplay their concerns.

D. Do not make the diagnosis of "febrile seizures" in the field. This diagnosis cannot be made until other causes are excluded. An important cause of seizures in childhood is meningitis (also associated with a fever). Other forms of encephalitis, head trauma, and epilepsy must also be excluded.

E. If the diagnosis of meningitis is made in the patient at a later time, be sure to check with the receiving hospital concerning the need for prophylactic antibiotics for the prehospital providers. This is usually not necessary if there was no mucous membrane contact with the patient (e.g., mouth-to-mouth breathing).

PEDIATRIC TABLES

TABLE 3-1. APGAR SCORE

Observation	2	1	0
Appearance (color)	Pink	Pink body Blue limbs	Blue
Pulse (heart rate)	> 100	< 100	None
Grimace (reflex irritability)	Cough, sneeze	Grimace	Non-responsive
Activity (muscle tone)	Active	Flexion of extremities	Limp
Respirations	Good cry	Slow, irregular	None

Neurologic evaluation of the newborn is best accomplished by using the APGAR scoring system. This system, like the Glasgow Coma Scale for adults, shows a great deal of inter-observer reliability and also has some prognostic value. Healthy, normal infants usually score between 8 and 10, while infants scoring less than 7 require significant resuscitative efforts.

It is unlikely that most paramedics will deliver enough infants to easily score the newborns he or she encounters. The important point is to make the necessary observations. If these are made accurately, a numerical score can be derived later. Thus, it is important to note the *color* of the infant, his *heart* and *respiratory rate*. Note his *muscle tone* when he is picked up. Finally, when suctioning, note the *reflex irritability* when the catheter is placed into his nose and posterior pharynx. The APGAR score is usually noted at one minute and at five minutes after birth. If the baby is unstable the observations should be repeated every 5 minutes. *Do not delay resuscitation while trying to calculate the APGAR score.*

TABLE 3-2. NORMAL VITAL SIGNS IN THE PEDIATRIC AGE GROUP

Age	Pulse beats/min	Respirations rate/min	Blood Pressure systolic +/–20
Premature	150	30 – 40	N/A
Newborn	140	30 – 40	N/A
6 month	130	20 – 36	80 palp
1 year	125	20 – 30	90 palp
3 years	115	20 – 30	95 palp
5 years	100	18 – 24	95 palp
8–10 years	90	12 – 20	100 palp

TABLE 3-3. PEDIATRIC AIRWAY SIZES

Age	Oral Airway	Endotracheal Tube (uncuffed)	Suction Catheter
Preemie	00	2.5–3.0	5 French
Newborn	0	3.0–3.5	6 F
6 months	0–1	3.5	8 F
18 months	1	4.0	8 F
3 years	2	4.5	10 F
5 years	2–3	5.0	10 F
8 years	3	6.0 Cuffed	10 F
Older	4	6.5–7.0 Cuffed	12 F

TABLE 3-4. PEDIATRIC TREATMENT REFERENCE

Treatment	Solution		Administration
IV fluids	RL, NS or D5RL		20 ml/kg
Dextrose 25%	250 mg/ml		2 ml/kg
Naloxone	0.4 mg/ml		0.1 ml/kg
Defibrillation			2 joule/kg
Sodium Bicarbonate	0.5 mEq/ml 4.2% for infants 10 kg or less		2 ml/kg
	1.0 mEq/ml 8.4% for infants over 10 kg		1 ml/kg
Epinephrine	1:10,000 0.1 mg/ml	IV	0.1 ml/kg
	1:1,000 1 mg/ml	SQ ET	0.01 ml/kg 0.1 ml/kg
Atropine	0.1 mg/ml		0.2 ml/kg
Lidocaine	20 mg/ml		0.05 ml/kg
Diazepam	5.0 mg/ml		0.04 ml/kg
Albuterol	2.5 mg/3 ml		1.5 ml < 2 yrs 3.0 ml > 2 yrs

TABLE 3-5.   PEDIATRIC DRUG DOSES FOR CRITICAL CARE

Age	pounds	kilogram	Na Bicarb 1 mEq/ml	Epi 1:10,000	Atropine 0.1 mg/ml	Lidocaine 20 mg/ml	Narcan 0.4 mg/ml	Dextrose 250 mg/ml	Diazepam 5 mg/ml	Defib 2 joules/kg
Newborn	5 #	2.2 kg	2.2 ml*	0.2 ml	1 ml	0.1 ml	0.2 ml	4.4 ml*	0.09 ml	5 joules
	10 #	4.5 kg	4.5 ml*	0.4 ml	1 ml	0.2 ml	0.4 ml	9.0 ml*	0.18 ml	10 joules
6 months	15 #	6.8 kg	7 ml*	0.7 ml	1.4 ml	0.3 ml	0.7 ml	14 ml	0.27 ml	15 joules
1 year	20 #	9.0 kg	9 ml*	0.9 ml	1.8 ml	0.5 ml	0.9 ml	18 ml	0.36 ml	20 joules
	25 #	11.3 kg	11 ml	1.1 ml	2.3 ml	0.6 ml	1.1 ml	23 ml	0.45 ml	25 joules
2 years	30 #	13.6 kg	14 ml	1.4 ml	2.7 ml	0.7 ml	1.4 ml	27 ml	0.54 ml	30 joules
	35 #	15.9 kg	16 ml	1.6 ml	3.2 ml	0.8 ml	1.6 ml	32 ml	0.64 ml	35 joules
4 years	40 #	18.1 kg	18 ml	1.8 ml	3.6 ml	0.9 ml	1.8 ml	36 ml	0.72 ml	40 joules
	50 #	22.7 kg	23 ml	2.3 ml	4.5 ml	1.1 ml	2.3 ml	45 ml	0.92 ml	50 joules
8 years	60 #	27.2 kg	27 ml	2.7 ml	5.0 ml	1.4 ml	2.7 ml	27 ml**	1.08 ml	60 joules
	70 #	31.8 kg	32 ml	3.2 ml	5.0 ml	1.6 ml	3.2 ml	32 ml**	1.28 ml	70 joules
10 years	80 #	36.3 kg	36 ml	3.6 ml	5.0 ml	1.8 ml	3.6 ml	36 ml**	1.44 ml	80 joules
	90 #	40.9 kg	41 ml	4.1 ml	5.0 ml	2.0 ml	4.1 ml	41 ml**	1.64 ml	90 joules
12 years	100 #	45.5 kg	46 ml	4.6 ml	5.0 ml	2.3 ml	4.6 ml	46 ml**	1.82 ml	100 joules

*Dilute with equal part saline prior to administration
**Dextrose 50%

4

TRAUMA TREATMENT PROTOCOLS

MULTIPLE TRAUMA OVERVIEW

Specific information needed

A. Mechanism of injury:

    1. Cause, precipitating factors, weapons.

    2. Trajectories and forces involved to patient.

    3. Vehicular trauma – condition of vehicle, windshield, steering wheel, use of seatbelts.

    4. Helmet use if motorcycle or bicycle.

B. Patient complaints.

C. Initial position and level of consciousness of patient from witnesses, first responders.

D. Patient movement, treatment since injury.

E. Other factors such as drugs, medications, diseases.

Specific objective findings

A. Scene evaluation:

    1. Note potential hazard to rescuers and patient.

2. Identify number of patients. Organize triage if appropriate.

3. Observe position of patient, surroundings, probable mechanism, vehicle condition.

B. Patient evaluation – initial assessment in multiple trauma patients is performed at the same time as treatment.

Initial assessment and treatment
Wear gloves and eye protection.

A. Evaluate scene. Make area safe for rescuers and patient, call for back-up as needed.

B. Airway:

1. Open airway using jaw thrust maneuver, keeping neck in neutral alignment.

2. Use assistant to provide cervical stabilization while managing ABCs.

3. Clear the airway using finger sweep, suction as needed.

4. Use towel clip or hand to draw tongue and mandible forward if needed in patients with facial injuries.

C. Breathing:

1. Treat respiratory arrest with:

   a. Pocket mask or bag-valve-mask for initial ventilatory control.

   b. CPR as needed.

   c. Intubate (prefer orotracheal) with cervical stabilization after initial ventilation as above. Confirm position of the tube, ventilate and monitor during transport.

   d. If difficulty with intubation, consider Dual-lumen airway.

   e. If none of the above are effective due to severe facial injury or other factors, perform cricothyrotomy. Confirm position of the tube, ventilate and monitor.

2. Look for signs of partial obstruction – noisy breathing, exaggerated chest wall movements. If present:

   a. Suction and clear manually.

   b. Reposition jaw while protecting neck.

   c. Insert oral or nasal airway as needed.

3. If respiratory rate < 12/minute, > 20/minute or breathing appears inadequate:

   a. Apply supplemental O_2, support with pocket mask or bag-valve-mask.

   b. Consider intubation – nasotracheal or orotracheal with firm cervical stabilization to secure airway.

   c. Confirm position of the tube, ventilate and monitor.

4. Inspect chest for symmetrical rise, sucking wounds, flail segment. If indicated:

   a. Stabilize flail and cover sucking wounds. (See Chest Injury Protocol)

   b. If ventilations, which were initially effortless, become difficult after bagging, consider tension pneumothorax decompression.

5. Apply O_2, moderate flow (4–6 L/min), by mask or nasal cannula (high flow with mask for critical patients). Titrate to pulse oximetry > 90% if possible.

D. Circulation:

1. Control exsanguinating hemorrhage by direct pressure with clean dressing to wound. (If needed, add elevation or pressure points. Use tourniquet only in extreme situation.)

2. Check radial pulse – presence implies BP > 80 mm Hg systolic. If not present, check carotid or femoral pulse (presence implies BP > 60–70 mm Hg systolic).

3. Check pulse for quality (strong, weak), general rate (slow, fast, moderate).

4. Check skin color, temperature, and capillary refill.

5. Initiate CPR and transport if no pulses are present unless multiple casualty scene or prolonged transport make resuscitation impossible.

E. Disability:

   1. Check level of consciousness, briefly, for essential elements – AVPU.

     A Alert

     V Responds to Verbal stimuli

     P Responds to Painful stimuli

     U Unconscious

   2. Check pupils – round? reactive? equal?

F. Obtain Vital Signs if patient stable or adequately resuscitated.

G. Immobilize cervical spine when appropriate (relieve assistant performing manual stabilization).

H. Apply PASG to spine board and transfer patient to board.

I. *Extricate and transport rapidly* if patient has multiple injuries or abnormal respiratory, circulatory or neurologic status.

J. Treat hypovolemic shock en route:

   1. Elevate legs, keep patient warm.

   2. Inflate PASG per protocol.

   3. IV – volume expander (NS or RL), large bore, two sites:

     a. TKO if patient appears stable and systolic BP > 90.

     b. Wide open if significant signs of shock, 20 ml/kg, further fluids as directed.

   4. Stabilize and splint fractures.

   5. Dress wounds if time allows.

K. If patient stable:

   1. Perform secondary survey and full neurologic exam. Record list of patient's problems.

   2. With significant injury or potential for hypovolemia, start IV – volume expander (NS or RL), large bore, one or two sites, TKO.

   3. Stabilize and splint fractures.

4. Dress wounds if possible.

5. Reassess and treat patient for life-threats:

    a. Adequacy of airway, breathing.

    b. Emergent chest injuries:

        1. Flail section.

        2. Tension pneumothorax.

        3. Cardiac tamponade.

        4. Sucking chest wound.

    c. Monitor closely for signs of hypovolemia.

L. Recheck vital signs, neurologic status, and monitor cardiac rhythm enroute.

Specific precautions

A. Although the organization of assessment and management may seem complex, remember the basic principles to keep organized.

1. As with any critical patient, assess and manage life threatening impairment of:

    a. Airway

    b. Breathing

    c. Circulation

2. If patient unstable, transport urgently *(load and go)*.

3. If the patient is stable, assess for *potentially* life-threatening injuries (secondary survey) and manage them.

B. Serial vital signs and observations of neurologic status in the field are critical. Use a flow chart to help organize information and observe if patient is improving or deteriorating.

C. Direct pressure will control most external hemorrhage. Continued direct hand pressure during transport may be required. Elevation of the injured area can be useful. Compression of the proximal arterial pressure point can be used if these fail. A tourniquet is *rarely* required and may increase bleeding if improperly applied. Use a proximal BP cuff inflated to 200 mm Hg to minimize tissue damage as a final resort for uncontrolled extremity hemorrhage.

D. Even in the noncritical patient with significant injury, "stabilization in the field" does not occur. With major injuries, the very most that can be done is to buy time. If the initial bolus of fluids or PASG inflation resulted in improved vitals, do not become complacent. This patient frequently needs blood and an operating room to truly "stabilize" the traumatic process. Rapid transport is still of the highest priority.

E. Recent literature has questioned the value of rapid fluid infusion for patients with ongoing internal bleeding. There is at least some evidence that internal bleeding may be increased with the administration of fluids. The final answer is not available, but it may be prudent to consider maintaining the IVs at TKO if the patient is not in profound shock. The establishment of one or two IVs will remain a priority. It is important to have the lines available should the patient deteriorate or for the rapid administration of fluids and blood in the operating room after the bleeding has been controlled. The earlier those vessels are cannulated the greater the success rate.

F. PASG use has become increasingly controversial. Inflation should be performed only within regional guidelines.

ABDOMINAL TRAUMA

Specific information needed
A. Patient complaints.

B. For penetrating trauma – weapon, trajectory.

C. For auto – condition of vehicle, steering wheel, dash, – air bags deployed, speed, patient trajectory, seatbelts in use, (type – lap/shoulder).

D. Past history – medical problems, medications.

Specific objective findings
A. Observe – distention, bruising, entrance/exit wounds.

B. Palpate – areas of tenderness, guarding, pelvis stability to lateral and suprapubic compression.

C. Condition of vehicle and steering wheel.

Treatment
A. Stabilize life-threatening airway, breathing and circulatory problems first. Obtain vital signs.

B. Apply PASG to board before moving patient.

C. IV – volume expander (NS or RL), large bore, TKO if patient stable.

D. For penetrating injuries – cover wounds and evisceration with moist saline gauze to prevent further contamination and drying. Do not attempt to replace.

E. Observe carefully for signs of blood loss. If BP < 90 systolic or significant signs of shock:

   1. Inflate PASG per protocol. (If large evisceration, inflate legs only.)

   2. Second IV, large bore, volume expander, if possible.

   3. Administer fluid bolus, 20 ml/kg, further fluids as directed.

F. Monitor vital signs during transport.

Specific precautions
A. The extent of abdominal injury is difficult to assess in the field. Be very suspicious; with significant blunt trauma, injuries to multiple organs are the rule.

B. Patients with spinal cord injury or altered sensorium due to drugs, alcohol, or head injury may not complain of tenderness and may lack guarding in the presence of significant intra-abdominal injury.

C. Seatbelts, steering wheels, and other blunt objects may cause occult intra-abdominal injury which is not apparent until several hours after the trauma, particularly in children. You must consider forces involved to properly treat a trauma victim. (This does *not* mean seatbelts should not be worn – trajectory injuries are much more lethal!)

AMPUTATED PARTS

Specific information needed

A. History – time and mechanism of amputation, care for severed part prior to rescuer arrival.

B. Past history – medical conditions, bleeding tendencies, meds.

Specific objective findings

A. Vital signs. Other injuries. Blood loss at scene.

B. Structural attachments in partial amputations if identifiable.

Treatment

A. Control hemorrhage with direct pressure, elevation.

B. Resuscitate and treat airway, breathing, and circulatory problems.

C. If significant hypotension:

    1. Apply PASG per protocol for bleeding or shock.

    2. IV – volume expander (NS or RL), 20 ml/kg, then TKO or as directed.

D. Patient – gently cover stump with sterile dressing. Saturate with sterile saline. Cover with dry dressing. Elevate.

E. Severed part – Wrap in sterile gauze, preserving all amputated material. Moisten with sterile saline. Place in water-tight container in cooler with ice (do not freeze).

F. Consult base for instruction on optimum transport destination.

Specific precautions

A. Partial amputations should be dressed and splinted in alignment with extremity to ensure optimum blood flow. Avoid torsion in handling and splinting.

B. Do not use *dry* ice to preserve severed part.

C. Control all bleeding by direct pressure only to preserve tissues. The most profuse bleeders may occur in partial amputations, where cut vessel ends cannot retract to stop bleeding. Avoid tourniquet if at all possible. Never clamp bleeding vessels.

D. Many factors enter into the decision to attempt reimplantation (age, location, condition of tissues, etc). Treatment decisions cannot be made until the patient and part have been examined by the specialist – and may not be made at the primary care hospital. Try to help the family and patient understand this and don't falsely elevate hopes.

CHEST INJURY

Specific information needed

A. Patient complaints – chest pain (type), respiratory distress, neck pain, other areas of injury.

B. Mechanism – amount of force involved, particularly deceleration, speed of impact, seatbelt use, type.

C. Penetrating trauma – size of object, caliber of bullet.

D. Past medical history – medications, medical problems.

Specific objective findings

A. Observe – wounds, air leaks, chest movement, neck veins.

B. Palpate – tenderness, crepitus, tracheal position, tenderness on sternal compression, pulse pressure.

C. Auscultate – breath sounds, heart sounds (quality).

D. Surroundings – weapons, vehicle, steering wheel condition.

Treatment

A. Clear and open airway. Stabilize neck.

B. Assist breathing if patient is apneic or respirations depressed.

C. Apply O_2, high flow (10–15 L/min) by mask. Titrate to pulse oximetry > 90% if possible.

D. Control exsanguinating hemorrhage with direct pressure.

E. If penetrating injury present, transport rapidly with further stabilization en route.

F. For open chest wound with air leak, use vaseline-type gauze occlusive dressing, plastic wrap or aluminum foil taped on three sides only, to allow air to escape but not enter the chest.

G. Observe chest for paradoxical movements. Treat lateral flail segment by splinting with sandbags or bags of IV fluid. Use hand pressure to sternum or other areas of the chest to minimize abnormal movement. If chest cannot be adequately stabilized by those means, consider intubation and positive pressure ventilation.

H. IV – volume expander (NS or RL), large bore, TKO.

I. Obtain baseline vital signs, neurologic assessment.

J. Evaluate neck veins and blood pressure:

    1. If neck veins flat and patient's BP < 90, transport rapidly and treat hypovolemia en route:

        a. Consider fluid bolus of 20 ml/kg, further fluids as directed.

        b. Monitor cardiac rhythm.

    2. If patient BP < 90, neck veins distended, also transport rapidly, and consider:

        a. Tension pneumothorax if respiratory status markedly deteriorating with clinical findings of pneumothorax:

            1. Release dressings on open chest wounds.

            2. Consider needle decompression.

        b. Pericardial tamponade if mechanism of injury suspicious (*may* have distant heart sounds and narrow pulse pressure):

            1. *Consider PASG inflation.

            2. *Consider fluid bolus of 20 ml/kg.

        c. Cardiac contusion with typical ischemic chest pain or severe chest wall contusion:

            1. Monitor cardiac rhythm.

            2. *Consider cautious fluid bolus of 10 ml/kg en route or as directed.

            3. *Lidocaine, 1 mg/kg, IV for significant PVCs.

    3. If BP > 90:

        a. Complete secondary survey.

        b. If significant injury present:

            1. Second IV, volume expander (NS or RL), large bore, TKO.

            2. Monitor cardiac rhythm enroute.

    3. *Lidocaine, 1 mg/kg, IV for significant PVCs.

  c. Bandage and splint if appropriate.

K. Immobilize impaled objects in place with dressings to prevent movement. If necessary transport sitting up or prone.

L. Monitor vitals and level of consciousness every five minutes.

Specific precautions

A. Chest trauma is treated with difficulty in the field and prolonged treatment before transport is *not* indicated. If patient is critical, transport rapidly and avoid treatment of nonemergent problems at the scene. Penetrating injury particularly should receive immediate transport with minimal intervention in the field.

B. Consider medical causes of respiratory distress such as asthma, pulmonary edema or COPD that have either caused trauma or been aggravated by it. Consider MI in single car crash.

C. Chest injuries sufficient to cause respiratory distress are commonly associated with significant blood loss. Look for hypovolemia.

EXTREMITY INJURIES

Specific information needed

A. Mechanism of injury, direction of forces, if known.

B. Areas of pain or limited movement.

C. Treatment prior to arrival – reduction of open or closed fracture, movement of patient.

D. Past medical history – medications, medical illnesses.

Specific objective findings

A. Vital signs.

B. Observe – localized swelling, discoloration, angulation, lacerations, exposed bone fragments, loss of function, guarding.

C. Palpate – tenderness, crepitus, instability, quality of distal pulses, sensation.

D. Note estimated blood loss at scene.

Treatment

A. Treat airway, breathing, and circulation as first priorities.

B. Immobilize cervical spine when appropriate.

C. Examine for additional injuries to head, face, chest, and abdomen. Treat problems with higher priority first.

D. If patient unstable, transport rapidly, treating life-threatening problems en route. Splint patient by securing to long board to minimize fracture movement.

E. If patient stable, or isolated extremity injury exists:

1. Check distal pulses and sensation prior to immobilization of injured extremity.

2. Apply sterile dressing to open fractures. Note carefully wounds that appear to communicate with bone, and initial position of bone in wound.

3. Splint areas of tenderness or deformity – apply gentle traction throughout treatment and try to immobilize the joint above and below the injury in the splint.

114

4. Reduce fractures (including open fractures) by applying gentle axial traction if indicated:

   a. To restore circulation distally.

   b. To immobilize adequately.

5. Check distal pulses and sensation after reduction and splinting.

6. Elevate simple extremity injuries. Apply padded ice if time and extent of injuries allow.

7. Monitor circulation (pulse and skin temperature), sensation, and motor function distal to the site of injury during transport.

Special precautions

A. Patients with multiple injuries have a limited capacity to recognize areas which have been injured. A patient with a femur fracture may be unable to recognize that he has other areas of pain. Be particularly aware of injuries proximal to the obvious ones (e.g., a hip dislocation with a femur fracture, or a humerus fracture with a forearm fracture).

B. Do not use ice or cold packs directly on skin or under air splints, pad with towels or leave cooling for hospital setting.

C. Do not attempt to reduce dislocations in the field. The only reasonable exception is a dislocated patella – if the diagnosis is clear and transport time is greater than 5 minutes – reduce dislocation by gently straightening the leg (after pain medication, if possible). Splint all dislocations in the position of comfort.

D. Fractures do not necessarily lead to loss of function. Impacted fractures may cause pain but little or no loss of function.

E. Do not allow severely angulated, open, bloody fractures to distract you from a less obvious pneumothorax with respiratory distress. Extremity injuries benefit from appropriate care, but are of low priority in a multiple-injured patient. Quick stabilization with a long board and generous taping is ample for the seriously injured patient.

F. Fractures near joints may become more painful and circulation may be lost with attempted reduction. If this occurs, stabilize the limb in the position of most comfort and with the best distal circulation.

FACE AND NECK TRAUMA

Specific information needed
A. Mechanism of injury – impact of steering wheel, windshield, or other objects. Clothesline-type injury to face or neck.

B. Management before arrival by bystanders, first responders.

C. Patient complaints – areas of pain, trouble with vision, hearing, neck pain, abnormal bite.

D. Past medical history – medications, medical illnesses.

Specific objective findings
A. Vital signs.

B. Airway – jaw or tongue instability, loose teeth, vomitus or blood in airway, other evidence of impairment or obstruction.

C. Neck – tenderness, crepitus, hoarseness, bruising, swelling.

D. Blood or drainage from ears, nose.

E. Level of consciousness, evidence of head trauma.

F. Injury to eyes, lid laceration, blood anterior to pupil, abnormal pupil, abnormal globe position or softness.

Treatment
A. Control airway:

1. Open airway using jaw thrust, keeping neck in alignment with manual stabilization.

2. Use finger sweep to remove teeth and other solid obstructions.

3. Suction blood and other debris.

4. Stabilize tongue and mandible with chin lift, manual traction or towel clip to tongue to keep posterior pharynx open as needed.

5. Note evidence of laryngeal injury and transport immediately if signs present.

6. With isolated facial injury, place patient prone or sitting up and leaning forward to ensure airway as needed.

7. Intubate if bleeding severe or airway cannot be maintained otherwise. Avoid nasotracheal intubation with mid-face trauma. If using orotracheal approach, ensure cervical stabilization to prevent neck extension. Confirm tube position immediately after intubation.

8. If intubation cannot be performed due to severe facial injury, attempt to manage with suctioning and supportive care. Consider dual-lumen airway.

9. If necessary, consider cricothyrotomy. Confirm tube position immediately after procedure.

B. Support breathing as needed. If mask fit cannot be maintained because of trauma, consider intubation or cricothyrotomy.

C. O_2, high flow (10–15 L/min). Titrate to pulse oximetry > 90% if possible.

D. Stop hemorrhage. Check pulse and circulation.

E. IV – volume expander (NS or RL), large bore:

1. TKO if stable.

2. With signs of shock, administer 20 ml/kg fluid bolus, further fluids as directed.

F. Immobilize cervical spine (relieve assistant performing cervical stabilization).

G. Obtain vital signs, assess neurologic status.

H. Complete secondary survey if no life-threatening injuries present.

I. Cover injured eyes with protective shield or cup – avoid pressure or direct contact to eye.

J. Do not attempt to stop free drainage from ears, nose. Cover lightly with dressing to avoid contamination.

K. Transport avulsed teeth with the patient. Keep moist in saline-soaked gauze.

L. If airway secured and patient stable, splint fractures and manage nonemergent injuries at scene or en route.

M. Monitor airway closely during transport for development of obstruction or respiratory distress. Suction and treat as needed.

Specific precautions

A. Fracture of the larynx should be suspected in patients with respiratory distress, abnormal voice, and history of direct blow to neck from steering wheel, rope, fence, wire, etc. Both intubation and needle cricothyrotomy may be unsuccessful in the patient with a fractured larynx and attempts may precipitate respiratory arrest. Transport rapidly for definitive treatment, if you suspect this potentially lethal injury. Do not attempt intubation or cricothyrotomy unless the patient arrests.

B. Airway obstruction is the primary cause of death in persons sustaining head and face trauma. Meticulous attention to suctioning, and stabilization of tongue and mandible may be the most important treatment rendered.

C. Remember that the apex of the lung extends into the lower neck and may be injured in penetrating injuries of the lower neck, resulting in pneumothorax or hemothorax.

D. Do not be concerned with contact lens removal in the field. The safest place for lenses is in the eye.

HEAD TRAUMA

Specific information needed

A. History – mechanism of injury, estimate of force involved, helmet worn with motorcycle or bicycle.

B. History since injury – loss of consciousness (duration), change in level of consciousness, memory loss for events before and after trauma, movement (spontaneous or performed by bystanders).

C. Past history – medications (insulin particularly), medical problems, seizure history.

Specific objective findings

A. Vital signs (note respiratory pattern and rate).

B. Neurologic assessment, including pupils, response to stimuli and Glasgow Coma Scale observations.

Glasgow Coma Score

Eye opening

None	1
To pain	2
To speech	3
Spontaneously	4

Best verbal response

None	1
Garbled sounds	2
Inappropriate words	3
Disoriented sentences	4
Oriented	5

Best motor response

None	1
Abnormal extension	2
Abnormal flexion	3
Withdrawal to pain	4
Localizes pain	5
Obeys commands	6

Total =
(15 points possible)

119

C. External evidence of trauma – contusions, abrasions, lacerations, bleeding from nose, ears.

Treatment

A. Assess airway and breathing. Treat life-threatening difficulties (see Trauma Overview). Use assistant to provide cervical stabilization while managing respiratory difficulty.

B. Control hemorrhage. Stop scalp bleeding with direct pressure if possible. Continued pressure may be needed.

C. Apply O_2, moderate flow (4–6 L/min), by mask or nasal cannula (high flow by mask for seriously injured patients). Titrate to pulse oximetry > 90% if possible.

D. Obtain initial vital signs, neurologic assessment, including Glasgow Coma Score.

E. If unconscious, or Glasgow Coma Score < 11:

   1. Assist ventilations.

   2. Consider intubation. If time allows administer lidocaine, 1.5 mg/kg IV, 1 minute prior to intubation.

   3. Hyperventilate at 20–30 breaths per minute.

F. Immobilize cervical spine (relieve assistant performing manual stabilization).

G. Immobilize patient on spine board (or other firm surface). Apply PASG to board prior to moving patient.

H. Secure patient to board following transfer. Be prepared to tilt for vomiting.

I. *Transport rapidly* if patient has multiple injuries, or unstable respiratory, circulatory, or neurologic status.

J. If BP < 90 mm Hg systolic and signs of hypovolemic shock are present, initiate treatment en route:

   1. Elevate legs, keep patient warm.

   2. Inflate PASG per protocol. Titrate to patient condition.

   3. IV – volume expander (NS or RL), large bore, wide open, 20 ml/kg, then TKO or as directed.

4. Consider bleeding sources (abdomen, pelvis, chest).

5. Stabilize and splint fractures and dress wounds if time allows.

K. If patient unconscious and showing signs of neurological deterioration (e.g., dilated pupil, rising BP, slowing pulse, posturing or decreasing GCS):

1. Hyperventilate at 20–30 breaths per minute.

2. *Consider furosemide, 20–40 mg IV.

3. *If transport time > 30 minutes, consider Foley catheter when diuretics have been administered.

L. If patient stable (respiratory, circulatory, neurologically):

1. IV – volume expander (NS or RL), large bore, TKO.

2. Complete secondary survey.

3. Splint fractures and dress wounds if time permits.

M. Monitor airway, vitals, and level of consciousness repeatedly at scene and during transport. *Status changes are important.*

Specific precautions

A. When head injury patients deteriorate, check first for airway, oxygenation and blood pressure. These are the most common causes of "neurologic" deterioration. If the patient has tachycardia or hypotension, look for hidden hypovolemia from associated injuries and do not blame the head injury.

B. The most important information you provide for the base physician is level of consciousness and its changes. Is the patient stable, deteriorating or improving?

C. Assume cervical spine injury in *all patients* with head trauma.

D. Restlessness can be a sign of hypoxia. Cerebral anoxia is the most frequent cause of death in head injury.

E. If active airway ventilation is needed, intubate and hyperventilate at 20–30/minute. *Hypoventilation* aggravates cerebral edema.

F. If patient is combative from head injury or hypoxia, consider use of morphine sulfate 2 mg IV, repeated every 5 minutes, titrated to reduce combativeness. The airway and C-spine can be more appropriately managed with a relaxed patient and the effects can be reversed at the receiving facility if desired. Administer cautiously *(slowly)* in hypovolemic patient.

G. Do not try to stop bleeding from nose and ears. Cover with clean gauze if needed to prevent further contamination.

H. Scalp lacerations can cause profuse bleeding, and are difficult to define and control in the field. If direct local pressure is insufficient to control bleeding, evacuate any large clots from flaps and large lacerations with sterile gauze and use direct hand pressure to provide hemostasis. If the underlying skull is unstable, pressure should be applied to the periphery of the laceration over intact bone.

SHOCK: TRAUMATIC

Specific information needed
A. Mechanism of injury – position, forces, speed, trajectory.

B. Patient complaints – thirst, dizziness, weakness, chest pain, trouble breathing.

C. Car – steering wheel and vehicle condition, seatbelt use and type.

D. Past medical history – medications, medical illnesses.

Specific objective findings
A. Vital signs – pulse > 120 (bradycardia or normal pulse rate may occur in some patients), BP < 90 systolic.

B. Mental status – mania or apathy, confusion, restlessness.

C. Skin – flushed, constricted, sweaty, cool or warm, color.

D. Signs of blunt injury or bleeding – flank hematoma, chest or abdominal wall contusion.

E. Jugular veins – flat or distended.

Treatment
A. Assess airway and breathing, treat life-threatening difficulties (see Trauma Overview). Use assistant to provide cervical stabilization while managing ABCs.

B. Control hemorrhage by direct pressure with clean dressing to wound. (If needed, add elevation, pressure points, tourniquet only in extreme situation.)

C. Obtain initial vital signs, neurologic assessment, including Glasgow Coma Score.

D. Immobilize cervical spine as appropriate, (relieve assistant performing cervical stabilization).

E. O_2, high flow (10–15 L/min). Titrate to pulse oximetry > 90% if possible.

F. Apply PASG to spine board and transfer patient to board.

G. IV – volume expander (NS or RL), large bore, TKO.

H. If BP < 90 systolic and neck veins flat, *transport rapidly* and treat shock en route:

1. Keep patient warm with blankets to prevent heat loss.

2. Raise legs 10–12 inches.

3. Inflate PASG per protocol. Titrate to patient condition.

4. Consider fluid bolus of 20 ml/kg, or as directed.

5. Monitor cardiac rhythm.

6. Look carefully for possible sources of bleeding (abdomen, pelvis, chest, scalp, back).

I. If BP < 90 systolic and signs of cardiogenic shock (distended neck veins), *transport rapidly* and consider:

1. Tension pneumothorax if respiratory status markedly deteriorating, with clinical findings of pneumothorax:

    a. Release occlusive dressings on open chest wounds.

    b. Consider needle decompression.

2. Pericardial tamponade if wound suspect (*may* have distant heart sounds, narrow pulse pressure):

    a. *Consider PASG inflation.

    b. *Consider fluid bolus of 20 ml/kg.

3. Cardiac contusion with typical ischemic chest pain or severe chest wall contusion:

    a. Monitor cardiac rhythm.

    b. *Consider cautious fluid bolus of 10 ml/kg en route or as directed.

    c. Lidocaine, 1 mg/kg IV for significant PVCs.

J. If BP > 90, observe closely and transport with PASG applied but not inflated.

1. Perform secondary survey and record patient's problems.

2. Maintain IV at TKO rate.

3. Stabilize and splint fractures.

4. Dress wounds as time allows.

K. Recheck vital signs and neurologic status en route – at least every 5 minutes with unstable patient.

Specific precautions

A. Hypotension itself is a late sign of hypovolemic shock. Blood loss must be anticipated from the mechanism of injury. Often a patient may suddenly "go bad" if the subtle clues aren't noticed beforehand.

B. Hypertensive and elderly patients can have significant hypotension at higher pressures than 90 systolic. Look for the adrenergic signs – vasoconstriction, sweating, mental alterations, agitation. Treat the entire picture and not just the blood pressure.

C. Neurogenic shock is caused by relative hypovolemia as blood vessels lose tone from spinal cord injury. Treat as for hypovolemia, and if hypotension persists, consider occult blood loss as an additional cause of shock.

D. While most shock in the setting of trauma is hypovolemic, assessment and treatment priorities should be organized to include a check for possible "cardiogenic" causes which should be managed differently. Pericardial tamponade, tension pneumothorax, myocardial contusion are rare but should be considered!

E. Occasionally, pain or cardiac contusion will cause inappropriate bradycardia. Consider also if an MI or a primary dysrhythmia may have caused the trauma. Fluid resuscitation should be cautious. Pain medication may also normalize the pulse *if* there are no contraindications.

F. Another important and frequent cause of "relative" bradycardia (pulse < 100) in the face of hypovolemic shock is the patient on beta-blocker drugs (e.g., propranolol), who cannot respond to blood loss with a tachycardia. Patients with angina, prior MI, migraine, hypertension, dysrhythmias and other medical illnesses may be taking beta-blockers. Treatment is the same, but do not wait for the tachycardia!

G. Recent literature has thrown some doubt on the wisdom of administering a large fluid bolus to all trauma patients who present in shock. Particularly in the face of ongoing internal hemorrhage, patients may do better with IVs at TKO until the bleeding can be stopped in the OR.

SPINAL TRAUMA

Specific information needed
A. Mechanism of injury and forces involved. Be suspicious with falls, airplane crashes, decelerations, diving accidents.

B. Past medical problems and medications.

Specific objective findings
A. Vital signs, including neurologic assessment.

B. Level of sensory deficit. Presence of any evidence of neurologic function below level of injury. Priapism.

C. Physical exam with careful attention to organs or limbs which may not have sensation.

Treatment
A. Assess airway and breathing. Treat life-threatening difficulties. Use controlled ventilation for high cervical cord injury associated with abdominal breathing. Use assistant to provide cervical stabilization while managing ABCs.

B. Control hemorrhage. Stop scalp bleeding with direct pressure if possible. Continued manual pressure may be needed.

C. Apply O_2, moderate flow (4–6 L/min) by mask or nasal cannula (high flow by mask for seriously injured patients). Titrate to pulse oximetry > 90% if possible.

D. Obtain initial vital signs, neurologic assessment, including Glasgow Coma Score.

E. Immobilize cervical spine with firm cervical collar. Maintain stabilization manually until securely immobilized on spine board.

F. Immobilize thoracic and lumbosacral spine with spine board (or other firm surface). Apply PASG to board prior to moving patient if needed. Move patient as little as possible and always move as a unit.

G. Secure patient to board following transfer. Secure trunk first, then head, then extremities.

H. IV – volume expander (NS or RL), large bore, TKO.

127

I. If patient BP < 90 mm systolic and signs of hypovolemic shock:

1. Keep patient warm with blankets to prevent heat loss.

2. Raise legs (or foot of spine board) 10–12 inches.

3. Inflate PASG per protocol. Titrate to patient condition.

4. Examine for possible sources of bleeding (abdomen, pelvis, chest, scalp, back).

5. Administer fluid bolus of 20 ml/kg or as directed.

J. If transport or extrication prolonged, contact base to consider *NG tube with intermittent suction using large syringe.

K. Mark level of sensory deficit gently with pen on patient's skin to facilitate monitoring.

L. Monitor airway, vitals, and neurologic status frequently at scene and during transport.

Specific precautions

A. Be prepared to tip entire board on side if patient vomits (patient must be secured to spine board or scoop stretcher –wide tape or straps anchored to both sides of board preferred).

B. Neurogenic shock is likely with significant spinal cord injury. Raise the foot of the spine board or legs only, whichever is easier logistically. Be sure respirations remain adequate.

C. If hypotension is unresponsive to simple measures, it is likely due to other injuries. Neurologic deficits make these other injuries hard to evaluate. Cord injury above the level of T-8 removes tenderness, rigidity, and guarding as clues to abdominal injury.

D. The patient with spinal trauma and normal neurologic function or only a partial deficit should not be treated more casually than the patient with a complete deficit. This is the patient who can benefit most from your conscientious splinting efforts and protection from further injury.

E. Spinal immobilization for patients with primarily penetrating trauma is rarely necessary. Consider immobilization when there is an apparent neurological deficit, an impaled foreign body, or other indication of specific cord damage.

SPECIAL TRAUMA PROBLEMS

Certain trauma situations call for assessment and treatment that goes beyond the standard treatment given for the patient's presenting complaints and injury. Treatment of physical injuries should be as listed in the protocols, but the following special considerations should be noted:

SEXUAL ASSAULT

A. History should not be more extensive than necessary from a medical standpoint. Legal and psychological details are best left to persons who will be able to use that information, follow it up with appropriate actions, and provide ongoing support to the patient.

B. You can, however, help with the patient's psychological needs. Do not judge the victim, who already feels debased, worthless, and guilty, no matter how blameless. Allow the patient as much freedom of choice in dealing with the medical community as possible. Do as little controlling as possible – let the patient control any aspects of care that he or she can. ("We need to start an IV. Would you like that in your left arm or your right?")

C. Remember that the radio waves are public. Particularly with sexual assault victims, refrain from names and details.

D. There may be hesitancy on the part of the victim to accept assistance from the same sex as the assailant. If an attendant of the other sex is available, it may be preferable to allow that attendant to treat. Be aware, however, that this can be a chance to revive faith in the other sex. Allow the patient to choose how interactive he or she would like to be.

E. You should encourage the victim to leave the same clothes on and not to bathe before coming to the hospital. This goes against a victim's instincts at the time but will help preserve legal evidence.

F. Encourage the victim to seek treatment even if reluctant to call the police and initiate legal action. There is still important medical treatment that can be offered, and the hospital staff or crisis counselor may allow the patient a better understanding of legal choices.

CHILD ABUSE/NEGLECT

A. Observe child for evidence of other injury, healing old wounds, multiple bruises. Also note how child relates to adults, physical and emotional relations within family unit.

B. Although some injuries, such as cigarette burns, are characteristic of child abuse, most abuse injuries are similar to many other injuries.

Suspicious scenarios include:

1. Injured child without obvious mechanism. Injuries which do not match story or stories which are inappropriate to the child's age.

2. Delay in seeking treatment.

3. Blame on third party.

4. Multiple different stories.

5. History of multiple previous episodes of trauma.

C. Don't accuse or judge. Observe, and share your observations with appropriate authorities. This is an instance where your skilled powers of observation in the field, and your ability to be discreet and to keep an open mind are most needed.

D. If abuse is suspected, transport the child, even if the injuries themselves do not warrant it. The same child may even be admitted for minor injuries to provide sufficient time to assess the situation and prevent serious injury or death in the future.

PREGNANT TRAUMA PATIENT

A. *Avoid supine positioning* in obviously pregnant patient. Pressure from the uterus on the inferior vena cava prevents venous return to the heart, and can result in severe hypotension. Turn patient to side (preferably left) or use your hands to hold uterus off central abdominal vessels.

B. Blunt abdominal trauma is difficult to evaluate because the abdominal exam is unreliable. Deceleration forces can cause placental separation. Seatbelts should be worn, but lap belts should be low, next to the pelvis, and fit snugly (more injuries still occur due to lack of seatbelt than are caused by them). All obviously pregnant patients should be transported for close evaluation and observation.

C. Think of eclampsia as a possible cause of injury in the pregnant trauma victim with altered mental state, seizures, or *hyper*tension.

D. Pregnancy alters normal vital signs as well as response to hypovolemia. Normal blood volume will be markedly increased at term. Normal BP will be lower with pulse slightly increased. Changes with hypovolemia are often delayed. Anticipate potential problems. Apply PASG and *inflate legs only* if needed.

E. The fetus is much more sensitive to hypoxia and hypovolemia than the mother. For this reason, O_2 should always be applied and treatment for blood loss should begin before hypotension becomes evident.

TRAUMA ARREST

A. Blunt trauma arrest – Confirm no respirations, no pulse. If there appears to be any chance of resuscitation (report of recent respiration, pulse, or movement, no apparent injury that would be incompatible with life):

1. Open airway, ventilate with bag-valve-mask.

2. Intubate to secure airway.

3. Needle decompression of chest if suspected tension pneumothorax.

4. Contact base to consider terminating efforts if no response and transport time significant.

B. Penetrating trauma arrest – Confirm no respirations, no pulse. If there appears to be any chance of resuscitation:

1. Open airway, ventilate with bag-valve-mask.

2. Extricate and begin *rapid transport* if within 20 minutes of hospital for definitive care.

3. Intubate to secure airway.

4. Needle decompression of chest if suspected tension pneumothorax.

5. IV – volume expander (NS or RL), wide open.

6. Contact base to consider terminating efforts if no response and longer than 20 minute transport to definitive care.

ENVIRONMENTAL TREATMENT PROTOCOLS

BITES AND STINGS

Specific information needed
A. Type of animal. Time of exposure.

B. Symptoms

   1. Local – pain, stinging.

   2. Generalized –nausea, weakness, itching, trouble breathing, dizziness, muscle cramps.

C. History of previous exposures, allergic reactions.

Specific objective findings
A. Identification of spider, bee, marine animal if possible.

B. Local signs – erythema, swelling, heat in area of bite.

C. Systemic signs – hives, wheezing, respiratory distress, abnormal vital signs.

Treatment

Snakes   See Snake Bites, page 151.

Spiders and scorpions
A. Ice for comfort.

B. Bring in spider if captured or if dead for accurate identification.

C. Transport for observation if systemic signs and symptoms present.

Bees and wasps
A. Remove sting mechanism. Try not to squeeze venom sac if this remains on stinger.

B. For at-home first aid – a paste of water and meat tenderizer (containing papain) can be applied for local symptomatic relief.

C. Observe patient for signs of systemic allergic reaction. Transport rapidly if needed. Treat anaphylaxis per protocol.

D. If patient has allergy kit, contact base to consider administration to patient as appropriate.

E. Transport all patients with systemic symptoms or history of systemic symptoms from prior bites.

Marine animals
A. Remove victim from water.

B. Treat airway, breathing, or other problems from water aspiration.

C. Assess and treat allergic reactions per protocol.

D. To prevent further contamination:

    1. Remove any stingers that can be easily lifted off (surgical removal is sometimes necessary).

    2. Remove nematocysts (from jellyfish, etc.) without squeezing or discharging.

        a. Wash with sea water (not fresh water).

        b. Pour alcohol (or vinegar) over area. Continue until pain relieved. May take 15–30 minutes.

        c. Dust cysts with flour, baking soda, talcum powder, or shaving cream, then gently scrape off remaining cysts.

E. For fish bites or stings, apply very warm water to skin for 15–30 minutes until pain relieved.

F. IV, volume expander (NS or RL), TKO if severe contamination has occurred. *Administer morphine sulfate, 2–4 mg IV, repeat as needed to total of 0.2 mg/kg for pain relief.

G. Transport patients with severe symptoms of envenomation or history of generalized allergic reaction.

Specific precautions
A. For all types of bites and stings, the goal of prehospital care is to prevent further inoculation and to treat allergic reactions.

B. Each region may need specific further protocols dependent on the exact type and severity of offending creatures in the area.

C. Alcohol inactivates the toxins in nematocysts of jellyfish and other coelenterates. Alcohol products include rubbing alcohol, perfume, liquor (at least 40%), or aftershave lotion.

D. Allergy kits consist of injectable epinephrine and oral antihistamine, and are prescribed for persons with known systemic allergic reactions. Prehospital care personnel still need to contact the resource hospital, even if assisting the patient with their own medication.

E. About 60% of patients who have experienced a generalized reaction to a bite or sting in the past will have a similar or more severe reaction upon reinoculation. Thus, although it is not inevitable, this group of patients must be considered at high risk for anaphylaxis. In addition, a small group of patients will have anaphylaxis as a "first" reaction.

F. Time since envenomation is important. Anaphylaxis rarely develops more than 60 minutes after inoculation.

BURNS

Specific information needed

A. History of injury – time elapsed since burn. Was patient in a closed space with steam or smoke? Electrical contact? Loss of consciousness? Accompanying explosion, falls, toxic fumes?

B. Past history – prior cardiac or pulmonary disease, medications?

Specific objective findings

A. Vital signs.

B. Extent of burns – description or diagram of areas involved (Figures 5-1 and 5-2) (during long transports only). Have diagrams ready to draw on.

C. Depth of burns – superficial – erythema only.
significant – blistered or charred areas.

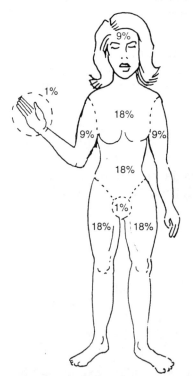

Figure 5-1. Burn – adult

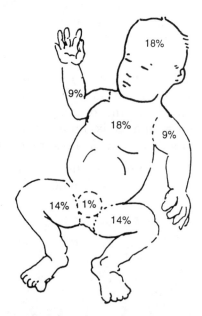

Figure 5-2. Burn – baby

D. Evidence of CO poisoning or other toxic inhalation – altered mental state, headache, vomiting, seizure, coma.

E. Evidence of inhalation burns – respiratory distress, cough, hoarseness, singed nasal or facial hair, soot or erythema of mouth.

F. Entrance and exit wounds for electrical burns.

G. Associated trauma.

Treatment

Thermal burn

A. Remove clothing which is smoldering or which is nonadherent to the patient.

B. O_2, high flow (10–15 L/min), mask with non-rebreathing bag, if indications of respiratory burns, toxic inhalation, or significant flame or smoke exposure. Titrate to pulse oximetry > 90% if possible.

C. Assess and treat for associated trauma (blast or fall).

D. Remove rings, bracelets, and other constricting items.

E. If significant burn is moderate-to-severe (over 15% of body surface area), cover wounds with dry clean dressings – use wet dressings only if skin still smoldering.

F. Use cool, wet dressings in smaller burns (less than 15%), for patient comfort.

G. If more than 30% significant burn and transport time > 30 minutes, contact base to consider:

1. Optimum destination hospital.

2. IV – volume expander (NS or RL), TKO or by amount of burn. Contact base for rate.

3. *Morphine sulfate, 2–4 mg, for pain relief. May repeat every 3 minutes, not to exceed 0.2 mg/kg.

H. Transport, monitoring vital signs.

Inhalation injury

A. O_2, high flow (10–15 L/min), using mask with non-rebreathing reservoir bag during full time of transport. Pulse oximetry may not be accurate with inhalation injuries – CO will give a falsely high pulse oximetry reading in spite of severe functional hypoxia.

B. Be prepared to ventilate or assist if respirations inadequate.

C. Consider need for early intubation.

D. Monitor cardiac rhythm.

Chemical burns

A. *Notify* HAZ-MAT Unit as soon as any chemical contamination is recognized. Protect rescuer from contamination. Wear appropriate gloves and clothing.

B. Remove all clothing and any solid chemical which might provide continuing contamination.

C. Assess and treat for associated injuries.

D. Decontaminate patient using running water for 15 minutes prior to transport.

E. Check eyes for exposure and rinse with free-flowing water for 15 minutes.

F. Evaluate for systemic symptoms which might be caused by chemical contamination. Contact base hospital for possible treatment.

G. Remove rings, bracelets, constricting bands.

H. Wrap burned area in clean, dry cloths for transport. Keep patient as warm as possible after decontamination.

I. Consult base or Poison Control Center (PCC) for special treatment or procedures as needed.

Electrical Injury

A. Protect rescuers from continued live electric wires.

B. Separate victim from electrical source only when area safe for rescuers.

C. Initiate CPR as needed. Defibrillation (per Cardiac Arrest protocol), *prolonged* respiratory support may be needed.

D. Immobilize cervical spine, assess for other injuries.

E. Monitor patient for possible dysrhythmias. Treat as per dysrhythmia protocol.

F. IV – volume expander (NS or RL), TKO or as directed.

Specific precautions
A. Leave blisters intact when possible.

B. Suspect airway burns in any facial burns or burns received in closed places. Edema may become severe, but not usually in the first hour. Avoid unnecessary trauma to the airway. Humidified O_2 is useful if available.

C. Death in the first 24 hours after burn injury is due to airway burns, fluid loss, or toxic inhalants (carbon monoxide or cyanide). Fluids are calculated on the basis of extent of *significant* burns, (i.e., those in which there is skin blistering or disruption).

D. Assume carbon monoxide poisoning in all closed space burns. Treatment is 100% O_2 continued for several hours, or hyperbaric oxygenation. In addition, other toxic products of combustion are more commonly encountered than realized. Many of these products will also give false pulse oximetry readings. Do not measure pulse oximetry in inhalation burns, since you may be falsely reassured in spite of ongoing *functional* hypoxia. Call base for special instructions if other toxic inhalations are suspected.

E. Consider MI as a cause of injury in firefighters who are burned. Consider suicide attempt as cause of burn, and child abuse in pediatric burns.

F. Lightning injuries can cause prolonged respiratory arrest. Prompt, continuous respiratory assistance (sometimes for hours to days) can result in full recovery.

G. Field decontamination of chemical exposures has been shown to significantly reduce extent of burn. It is rare to encounter a chemical which is not properly decontaminated by copious water. Unless a specific contraindication is known, do not waste time before initiating treatment to find out the specific culprit.

H. Oxygen may increase the vigor of combustion. Make sure all smoldering clothing is extinguished before placing in the presence of oxygen.

DECOMPRESSION/DIVING INJURY

Specific information needed
A. Symptoms

    1. Chest – pain, trouble breathing, cough.

    2. Joints – pain, cramps.

    3. CNS – headache, dizziness, fatigue.

B. Setting

    1. Underwater diving.

    2. Depressurization or inadequate pressurization while flying at high altitudes.

    3. Tunnel or deep excavation work.

    4. Air tank failure during dive.

    5. High altitude exposure (such as air flight) after scuba diving.

    6. Swimming with use of pressurized breathing equipment (scuba gear).

Specific objective findings
A. Decompression illness

    1. Cough, respiratory distress without pneumothorax.

    2. CNS – focal central or spinal deficits, confusion, seizures, coma.

    3. Cardiovascular – dysrhythmias, low BP.

    4. Skin – tenderness, mottling, red rash from bubble emboli.

B. Air embolism

    1. Pneumothorax, tension pneumothorax.

    2. Focal signs as above.

Treatment
A. Decompression illness

    1. Keep patient at complete rest in supine position.

    2. O_2, high flow (10–15 L/min), mask with reservoir bag.

3. IV – volume expander (NS or RL), large bore, TKO or as directed.

4. Contact base for optimum transport destination if decompression chamber exists locally.

B. Air embolism

1. Treat as above for decompression illness.

2. Observe for signs of tension pneumothorax and treat with rapid transport.

3. Consider needle decompression if indicated.

Specific precautions
A. Protocols will vary in different regions. In those areas where diving emergencies are seen commonly, procedures should be arranged in conjunction with military or other barotrauma specialists.

B. Decompression illness is secondary to formation of nitrogen bubbles in the bloodstream as atmospheric pressure decreases, and excess gas comes out of solution in the blood, usually during ascent from a dive or when using pressurized breathing apparatus. Air emboli occur when decreasing pressures cause air in the lungs to overexpand and rupture alveoli. In addition to lung damage, embolization of gas can cause a stroke-like picture from blocked flow in other distal arteries.

C. "Bends", the most common form of decompression illness, is caused by nitrogen bubbles in joints and bones, and usually occurs within 3 hours of surfacing. Though "bends" are extremely uncomfortable, they are not usually fatal. Patients with "bends" should be watched carefully, however, because other more serious forms of decompression illness can develop.

DROWNING/NEAR-DROWNING

Specific information needed
A. How long patient was submerged.

B. Fresh or salt water, degree of contamination, water temperature.

C. Diving accident. Water depth.

Specific objective findings
A. Vital signs.

B. Neurologic status – monitor on a continuing basis.

C. Lung exam – crackles or signs of pulmonary edema, respiratory distress.

Treatment
A. Clear upper airway of vomitus or large debris.

B. Start CPR if needed. Do not drain lungs prior to initiating ventilatory assistance except in sea-water victims.

C. Stabilize neck prior to removing from water if any suggestion of neck injury. Remove from water on back-board.

D. Suction as needed.

E. O_2, high flow (10–15 L/min), mask with non-rebreathing reservoir bag, regardless of condition.

F. If patient not awake and alert:

   1. Assist ventilation using pocket mask or bag-valve-mask.

   2. Intubate and apply positive pressure ventilation.

   3. IV – volume expander (NS or RL), TKO or as directed.

   4. *Consider sodium bicarbonate, 0.5 mEq/kg IV.

   5. Monitor cardiac rhythm during transport.

G. Transport patient, even if normal by initial assessment.

Specific precautions
A. Be prepared for vomiting. Patients should be secure on spine board for log-rolling to protect airway.

B. *All* near-drownings or submersions should be transported. Even if patients initially appear fine, they can deteriorate. Monitor closely. Pulmonary edema often occurs due to aspiration, hypoxia, and other factors. It may not be evident for several hours after near-drowning.

C. Beware of neck injuries – they often go unrecognized. Collar and backboard can be applied in the water if the patient is not yet on land.

D. If patient is hypothermic, defibrillation may be unsuccessful until the patient is rewarmed. Prolonged CPR may be needed. See Hypothermia Protocol.

HIGH ALTITUDE ILLNESS

Specific information needed
A. Present symptoms – headache, trouble breathing, confusion, fatigue, nausea.

B. Current and highest altitude, time at this altitude, duration of ascent.

C. Medical problems, medications, previous experience at altitude.

Specific objective findings
A. Vital signs.

B. Mental status – confusion, lack of coordination, coma.

C. Lungs – respiratory rate, distress, wet lung sounds, sputum (bloody or frothy).

Treatment
A. Put patient at rest, position of comfort.

B. O_2, high flow (10–15 L/min), by mask with non-rebreathing reservoir bag.

C. Reduce flow after 30 minutes to 1–2 L/min to conserve O_2 during long transports.

D. Suction as needed. Assist ventilations if patient has cyanosis, confusion, and poor respiratory effort.

E. Descend with patient at least 2,000–3,000 feet. If symptoms severe, use litter or personnel to carry patient.

F. IV – D5W, TKO, if conditions permit, or saline lock.

G. Monitor vitals during transport.

Specific precautions
A. Recognition of the problem is the most critical part of treating high altitude illness. While in the mountains, recognize symptoms which are out of proportion to those being experienced by the rest of the party – fatigue, or trouble breathing (particularly at rest).

B. The mainstay of treatment is descent from altitude. Even a loss of 2,000–3,000 feet makes enough difference in the O_2 content of air that symptoms may be relieved or stop progressing. Oxygen administration can also relieve symptoms and may allow more time for orderly evacuation.

C. In addition to the more common pulmonary edema, cerebral edema may occur, with confusion and a stroke-like picture with focal deficits. Treatment is the same.

D. Acute mountain sickness, the mildest form of illness during altitude adaptation, consists of fatigue, headache, poor sleeping *without* CNS or respiratory symptoms. Treatment is rest and hydration. This increases the body's time to acclimatize.

E. Commercial airlines pressurize cabins to a level approximately equivalent to 7,000–9,000 ft at cruising altitude. Persons with COPD, angina, or pneumothorax may experience problems with this level of oxygenation, much as they would visiting a city at that altitude.

F. Diuretics are not useful in treating high altitude pulmonary edema because the cause is excess capillary leakage of fluid rather than increased venous pressure. Some patients may be taking the diuretic acetazolamide, however, because of the indirect effects on acid-base balance.

G. When evaluating high altitude illness while in the mountains recreationally, do not be overly casual. Any party member with suspected acute mountain illness who is mentally confused or who has resting tachycardia or increased respiratory rate should be helped to descend without delay. Do not allow a hiker to "rest overnight" if symptoms are present at rest *or* if location is such that treatment with oxygen is not immediately available.

HYPERTHERMIA

Specific information needed
A. Patient age, activity level.

B. Medications – depressants, tranquilizers, alcohol, etc.

C. Associated symptoms – cramps, headache, orthostatic symptoms, nausea, weakness.

Specific objective findings
A. Vital signs, temperature – usually 104 degrees Fahrenheit (40 degrees Centigrade) or greater.

B. Mental status – confusion, coma, seizures, psychosis.

C. Skin flushed and warm – with or without sweating.

D. Air temperature and humidity, patient dress.

Treatment
A. Ensure airway.

B. O_2, moderate flow, 4–6 L/min. Titrate to pulse oximetry > 90%.

C. Remove clothing. Cool with water-soaked sheets. Ensure adequate air flow over patient for evaporative loss.

D. IV – volume expander (NS or RL), large bore:

    1. TKO if vital signs stable.

    2. Fluid bolus of 20 ml/kg, if signs of hypovolemia. Further fluids as needed.

E. Test blood for glucose level.

F. Administer dextrose 50%, 50 ml IV, in secure vein, if glucose level < 60 mg/dl.

G. Administer diazepam 5–10 mg IV for seizures.

H. Monitor cardiac rhythm.

I. Monitor vitals during transport.

Specific precautions
A. Heat *stroke* is a medical emergency. It is distinguished by altered level of consciousness. Sweating may still be present especially

in exercise-induced heat stroke. Other persons at risk for heat stroke are the elderly and persons on medications which impair the body's ability to regulate heat.

B. Differentiate heat *stroke* from – heat *exhaustion* (hypovolemia of more gradual onset), and heat *cramps* (abdominal or leg cramps). Be aware that heat exhaustion can progress to heat stroke.

C. Do not use wet sheets over patient without good air flow. They will tend to increase temperature by limiting evaporative loss.

D. Definitive cooling requires ice water baths and *careful* monitoring. *Do not let cooling in the field delay your transport.* Cool patient as possible while enroute.

HYPOTHERMIA AND FROSTBITE

Specific information needed
A. Length of exposure.

B. Air temperature, water temperature, winds, patient wet, or wet clothes.

C. History and timing of changes in mental status.

D. Medications – steroids, alcohol, tranquilizers, anticonvulsants, others.

E. Medical problems – diabetes, epilepsy, alcoholism, etc.

F. With local injury – history of thawing or refreezing?

Specific objective findings
A. Vital signs, mental status, shivering. (Prolonged observation for 1–2 minutes may be necessary to detect pulse, respirations.)

B. Temperature – rectal < 95 degrees Fahrenheit (35 degrees Centigrade) is significant. Note also current temperature of environment.

C. Evidence of local injury – blanching, blistering, erythema of extremities, ears, nose.

D. Cardiac rhythm.

Treatment

Generalized hypothermia
A. CPR if NO pulse or respirations. Prolonged CPR may be required. (If monitor present, no CPR if organized electrical activity present.)

B. O$_2$, moderate flow (4–6 L/min), warm, humidified if possible. Titrate to pulse oximetry > 90%.

C. Avoid unnecessary suctioning or airway manipulation.

D. Remove wet or constrictive clothes from patient. Wrap in blankets and protect from wind exposure.

E. IV – volume expander (NS or RL), large bore, TKO or as ordered. Solution should be warmed if possible. Do not start IV until patient is moved to transport vehicle.

F. Test blood for glucose level.

G. Dextrose 50%, 50 ml IV in secure vein if glucose level < 60 mg/dl or unable to test.

H. Consider naloxone, 2 mg IV for suspected narcotic toxicity.

I. Monitor cardiac rhythm. Attempt defibrillation, if appropriate, one time only.

J. Monitor vitals during transport.

Local (frostbite)
A. Remove wet or constricting clothing. Keep skin dry and protected from wind.

B. Do not allow the limb to thaw if there is a chance that limb may refreeze before evacuation is complete or if patient must walk to transportation.

C. Rewarm minor "frostnip" areas by placing in rescuer axilla or against trunk under clothing.

D. Dress injured areas lightly in clean cloth to protect from pressure, trauma or friction. Do not rub. Do not break blisters.

E. Maintain core temperature by keeping patient warm with blankets, warm fluids, etc.

F. Transport with frostbitten areas supported and elevated if feasible.

Specific precautions

Hypothermia
A. Shivering does not occur below 90 degrees Fahrenheit (32 degrees Centigrade). Below this the patient may not feel cold, and occasionally will even undress and appear vasodilated.

B. The heart is most likely to fibrillate below 85–88 degrees Fahrenheit (29.4–31 degrees Centigrade). Defibrillation should be attempted, but prolonged CPR may be necessary until the temperature is above this level.

C. ALS drugs should be used sparingly, since peripheral vasoconstriction may prevent entry into central circulation until temperature is restored. At that time a large bolus of unwanted drugs may be infused into the heart. Bradycardias are normal and should not be treated.

D. Any handling and airway manipulation may induce ventricular fibrillation in the hypothermic patient. Delay intubation if airway can be managed by less invasive means. If time permits, consider administration of prophylactic lidocaine, 1.5 mg/kg IV, approximately one minute prior to intubation.

E. If patient has even a faint pulse, organized monitor rhythm and occasional respirations, CPR is currently felt to be unnecessary. In general, even very slow rates are probably sufficient for metabolic demands, CPR is indicated for asystole and ventricular fibrillation, though the compression rate can be slower than usual (40/minute).

F. Patients who appear dead after prolonged exposure to cold air or water should not be pronounced "dead" until they have been rewarmed. Full recovery from hypothermia with undetectable vital signs, severe bradycardia, and even periods of cardiac arrest have been reported.

G. Rewarming should be accomplished with careful monitoring in a hospital setting whenever possible.

H. Early recognition of hypothermia is essential when exposed to cooling weather (either wet or cold). Death often occurs because the patient becomes apathetic, confused, and unable to help himself. When medical care is not readily accessible, rewarming may be attempted while someone goes for help. Place the patient with rescuer in sleeping bag and bundle with warm blankets.

Frostbite
A. Thawing is extremely painful and should be done under controlled conditions, preferably in the hospital. Careful monitoring, pain medication, prolonged rewarming, and sterile handling are required.

B. It is clear that partial rewarming, or rewarming followed by refreezing, is far more injurious to tissues than delay in rewarming or walking on a frozen extremity to reach help. *Do not rewarm prematurely*. Indications for field rewarming are few.

C. Warming with heaters or stoves, and rubbing with snow may further damage desensitized tissue, and should not be used. Drinking alcohol and other methods of stimulating the circulation are also dangerous.

SNAKE BITES

Specific information needed
A. Type of snake.

B. Time of bite.

C. Prior first-aid by patient or friends.

D. Symptoms – paresthesias, peculiar or metallic taste sensations, local pain; later – chills, headache or nausea, numbness or tingling of mouth, tongue, other areas.

Specific objective findings
A. Bite wound – location, configuration (1, 2, or 3 fang marks, entire jaw imprint, none).

B. Signs of envenomation – local edema or swelling, later signs may include fever, vomiting, discoloration around the fang site, hypotension.

Treatment
A. Remove patient and rescuers from area of snake to avoid further injury.

B. Remove rings or other bands which may become tight with local swelling.

C. Immobilize bitten part as for a fracture.

D. Minimize venom absorption by keeping bite area still and patient quiet.

E. If signs of envenomation are present, apply light constricting band 1 inch wide, 2–3 inches proximal to bite. It should admit one finger under it with ease.

F. Transport promptly for definitive observation and treatment.

    1. *Do not use ice or refrigerants.*

    2. Do not make incisions or attempt to suction wound.

Specific precautions
A. Find out the specific poisonous snakes present in your region. Treatment varies; even with rattlesnakes there are regional

differences in size and potency of venom. If the snake is dead, bring it in for examination. Do not jeopardize fellow rescuers by attempting to "round it up." Be careful – a dead snake may still reflexively bite and envenomate.

B. At least 25% of poisonous snake strikes do not produce envenomation. Do not overtreat the patient who does not have symptoms.

C. Fang marks are characteristic of pit viper bites such as the rattlesnake, water moccasin, or copperhead which are native to North America. Jaw prints (without fangs) are more characteristic of nonvenomous species. However, do not overlook the less obvious bites of the coral snake with few local signs, but increased risk of systemic reaction – including confusion and respiratory arrest.

D. Small children and elderly persons are at greatest risk from poisonous bites. Treatment should be more aggressive for these patients.

E. Ice can cause serious tissue damage.

F. More dangerous problems can develop from uncontrolled incision of bite wounds than from envenomation itself. Current recommendations are to avoid incisions.

G. Exotic poisonous snakes, such as those found in zoos, have different signs and symptoms than those of pit vipers. Information should be obtained from zoo or Poison Control Center (PCC) for proper identification and treatment.

6

HAZARDOUS MATERIALS PROTOCOLS

INTRODUCTION

This chapter is exclusively for paramedics with additional training. This material is *not* covered in the national DOT training program. Additionally, the risks involved (to the paramedic) in caring for these patients are far greater than the average patient.

Our recommendation is that this chapter *only* be used by specially trained paramedics who work regularly with a Hazardous Materials Response Team. Those are the only personnel who will have adequate equipment, protective gear, and training to safely approach many of these patients. *Safety of the rescuer is of primary importance.* Unconscious or dead paramedics are no help to anyone!

It is critical for the average EMS responder to recognize a hazardous materials incident and notify the appropriate personnel. The following situations should raise suspicions of hazardous materials being involved:

A. Train derailments.

B. Vehicle related incidents involving Department of Transportation (DOT) placarded vehicles or labeled substances. Any incident involving a vehicle which is used for transporting goods that has a cargo suspected to be a hazardous material whether the vehicle is placarded or not.

C. Vehicle related incidents involving unknown loads or unusual containers including liquid and gas transporters.

D. Incidents involving unknown or suspicious substances which have spilled or leaked, including unknown odors.

E. Incidents involving storage areas which may contain hazardous materials.

F. Scenes with multiple victims becoming ill for unknown reasons.

G. Scenes involving explosions or explosive substances.

H. Incidents involving aircraft – "crop dusters" are particularly suspect.

I. School laboratories often contain a number of dangerous chemicals.

The circumstances listed above could prove a deadly trap to the eager first responder or EMT. Restrain yourself and notify the proper Hazardous Materials Unit or authorities, before further investigation. The appropriate response to the hazardous materials incident goes against every instinct of the prehospital care provider. You can't run in to rescue someone if you might be killed in the process, but it is extremely difficult to stand back and alert authorities when your usual approach is to run in. Mentally prepare yourself ahead of time. The urge to run in is not worth your life!

APPROACH TO HAZARDOUS MATERIALS (Figure 6-1)

Approach to scene

A. Prepare through familiarization with authorized Department of Transportation (DOT) placards, labels, 704 System, and observe site proximity for the presence of such labels.

B. Obtain a copy of the DOT Emergency Response Guidebook and become proficient using it. Keep this book available in the vehicle at all times. Do not rely on your memory.

C. Be suspicious of large trucks or tractor-trailers transporting goods even if placards are not visible. At buildings or locations with NFPA 704 placard, consider hazardous condition, prior to entering scene.

D. If any serious consideration of hazardous materials contamination, contact dispatch to request Hazardous Materials Response Team (HMRT), and other appropriate personnel and equipment. Await arrival of responding units prior to any advancement into the scene.

E. If dispatch information is received that a scene has hazardous materials involved or for any reason you suspect the presence of such materials *do not enter the scene!* The following guidelines should improve safety:

   1. Observe posted barriers *(do not cross the barrier tape!)*

   2. Approach uphill and upwind from the incident and only when requested or assisted by the HMRT or Incident Commander.

   3. For leaks from drums, small containers or tanks – maintain 600 to 800 feet distance.

   4. For large leaks or spills, maintain at least 1000 to 1500 feet distance.

   5. In the event of a fire involving hazardous materials, maintain $^{1}/_{2}$ to 1 mile distance.

F. An area should be established for staging ambulances as soon as possible. All crews and units shall stay in that area until advised by the HMRT or Medical Officer as designated by the Incident Command System (ICS).

HAZARDOUS MATERIALS INCIDENT

- HOT ZONE: Proper level of protective clothing and assigned task
- WARM ZONE: Operations area for assigned support functions
- COLD ZONE: Safe perimeter area that is monitored by response team and supported by police department
- DECON AREA: Area for decontamination of all equipment. This area provides decontamination provisions for personnel, equipment and victims

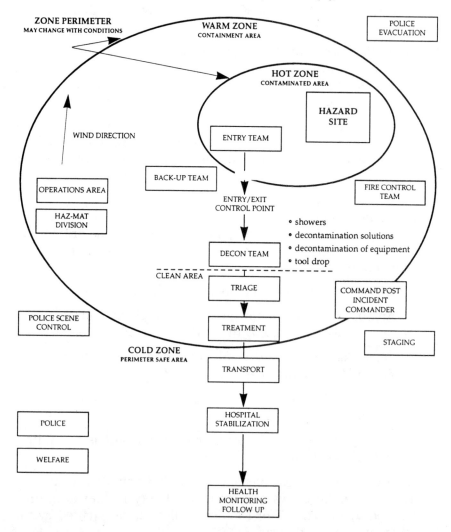

Figure 6-1. Hazardous Materials

Scene management

A. Once a "Hot Zone" is established, there should be only one entrance and exit into that area, which will be controlled by the HMRT exclusively.

B. A "Safety Perimeter" will be established at the outermost safe limits for the evacuation area. Only people directly involved with the incident will be admitted.

C. Keep non-contaminated people away from the incident scene or move them uphill and upwind, at a distance that is determined to be safe.

D. Avoid gaseous clouds, concentrations of vapor, and smoke.

E. Don't assume that if you can't see it or smell it – it is not harmful.

F. Keep contaminated victims away from noncontaminated people. A public address system may be necessary. Do not allow contaminated individuals, equipment, or materials to leave the "Hot Zone" until it is determined by the HMRT that it can be done safely.

G. Do not enter an area without permission from the HMRT (or IC) and the proper protective gear.

H. If you find yourself in a situation where you have been contaminated or you are within a "Hot Zone" on a Haz-Mat scene, back out to a safe position, but *do not leave the scene*. Isolate yourself from others and contact the HMRT for decontamination (decon) procedures.

I. Any information obtained about the material should be passed on to the HMRT and/or Haz-Mat Paramedic to be utilized in scene mitigation.

J. All members of HMRT should be medically evaluated and rehabilitated prior to exiting the scene. This will be managed by the Haz-Mat Paramedic and/or the Incident Commander.

K. *Beware of changing conditions (weather, fire size, or intensity, etc.). Be ready to retreat rapidly by way of predetermined egresses.*

Decontamination

A. When the HMRT dictates that the material involved requires proper decontamination, all victims must be decontaminated by going through the HMRT decon process prior to leaving the scene. *No patient should be transferred to the ambulance or emergency department until they have gone through this process.* Failure to complete this step could lead to numerous unneeded exposures and a compounding of an already serious problem.

B. All personnel involved with the decon process should be in proper protective equipment.

C. Prior to transport the receiving hospital must be notified of the situation, material involved, and that the patient has been through the decontamination process.

D. As soon as patient numbers, information on the material, and extent of exposure has been determined the Haz-Mat Paramedic or Medical Control Officer should notify the receiving hospital(s).

General Medical Approach

A. Protect rescuers

B. History

C. Patient assessment

    1. *Need for decontamination*

    2. Airway, breathing and circulation

    3. Level of consciousness and gag reflex

    4. Secondary survey

D. Generalized treatment

    1. *Decontamination*

    2. Assure airway, breathing and circulation

    3. Eye irrigation

    4. Supportive treatment – treat signs and symptoms

    5. Prevention of absorption

        a. *Decontamination*

        b. Induce emesis, perform lavage

        c. Charcoal

        d. Cathartic

E. Specific physiological antagonists

   1. Cyanide kit

   2. Atropine

   3. 2-PAM

   4. Methylene Blue

   5. Calcium gluconate

F. Assess and treat for other injuries, illnesses

ACETYL CHOLINESTERASE INHIBITORS

Source
A. Insecticides

Organophosphates

Tetraethylpyrophosphate (TEPP) Parathion Phorate Disulfoton Mevinphos	Highly toxic
Diazinon Coumaphos Chlorpyrofos Crufomate Trichlorfon	Moderately toxic
Malathion	Low toxicity

Carbamates

Aldicarb Carbofuran Tirpate	High toxicity
Aminocarb Befencarb Methomyl	Moderately toxic
Carbaryl	Low toxicity

B. Non insecticide carbamates

Physostigmine (Antilirium)
Neostigmine (Prostigmin)
Edrophonium (Tensilon)

C. Nerve gases – usually organophosphates

Clinical presentation
A. Early or mild exposure:

1. Fatigue, anorexia, nausea

2. Vertigo, weakness

3. Loss of concentration, blurred vision

B. Moderate to severe exposure:

   1. Muscarinic effects – miosis

      S – Salivation, increased secretions

      L – Lacrimation

      U – Urination

      D – Defecation, dyspnea, dysrhythmias

      G – GI distress – abdominal cramps, diarrhea

      E – Emesis

   2. Nicotinic effects – mydriasis

      M – Muscle twitching and cramps

      T – Tachycardia

      W – Weakness

      tH – Hypertension

      F – Fasciculations

   3. CNS effects – excitability, lethargy, seizures, coma

Treatment

A. Assure safety of rescuers.

B. Decontaminate.

C. Airway, protect as needed.

D. O_2, high flow (10–15 L/min). Titrate to pulse oximetry > 90%.

E. Suction as necessary.

F. IV – volume expander (NS or RL), TKO or as directed.

G. Administer atropine 2–4 mg IV, repeat every 2–5 minutes until bronchial secretions clear or signs of atropinization (hot, dry, flushed, or dilated pupils).

   Pediatric dose is 0.015 to 0.005 mg/kg IV, repeat if needed as above.

H. In organophosphate poisoning administer pralidoxime – 1 gm in 100 ml D5W over 15 minutes, may need to repeat to effect.

   Pediatric dose is 25 mg/kg administered over 15 minutes and repeated as necessary.

I. Observe for seizures or pulmonary edema and treat as necessary.

J. Transport as soon as possible.

Special notes

A. Organophosphates, carbamates, and nerve gas are absorbed rapidly through every route – oral, conjunctival, skin, or respiratory tract. Some act directly and very rapidly, others are toxic only after being metabolized and therefore the effects may be delayed.

B. Organophosphates and carbamates act as acetylcholinesterase inhibitors. Acetylcholinesterase is the enzyme that digests or incapacitates acetylcholine. Acetylcholine is the primary neurotransmitter for skeletal muscle, the parasympathetic nervous system, the preganglionic sympathetic nerve endings, and much of the central nervous system (CNS). With no enzyme to digest acetylcholine the nerve endings continually fire. The effects are described as "muscarinic" (parasympathetic nerve ending stimulation), "nicotinic" (striated muscle and sympathetic ganglia stimulation) and CNS stimulation.

C. When organophosphates and carbamates bind with acetylcholinesterase, it is initially reversible. The carbamates will spontaneously hydrolyze from the cholinesterase within 48 hours. Organophosphates will not spontaneously release, and in fact the binding is only reversible for 24–48 hours. After that time, if no antidote (pralidoxime) has been administered, the cholinesterase will be irreversibly destroyed.

CYANIDE

Source
A. Pest control
1. Vermicidal fumigant
2. Insecticide
3. Rodenticide
4. Soil sterilization
5. Coyote "gitter" traps

B. Industrial uses
1. Metal polish
2. Electroplating
3. Extracting silver and gold from ore
4. Photography
5. Chemical synthesis
6. Removing hair from hides

C. Fires
1. Wool
2. Silk
3. Polyurethanes
4. Polyacrylonitriles
5. Horsehair

D. Plants and fruit
1. Amygdalin (Laetrile)
2. Peach, cherry and apricot pits
3. Apple and pear seeds

E. Sodium nitroprusside

F. Cigarette smoke

G. Artificial nail removers (acetonitrile)

Clinical presentation

A. Early or mild exposure – odor of bitter almonds

   1. Respiratory – tachypnea, hyperpnea

   2. CNS – anxiety, confusion, vertigo, headache

   3. Cardiac – tachy or irregular pulse

   4. GI – nausea, vomiting

   5. Skin – flushed, hot and dry

B. Late or severe exposure

   1. Respiratory – gasping efforts then apnea

   2. CNS – seizures and coma

   3. Cardiac – bradycardia and cardiovascular collapse

Treatment

A. Assure safety of rescuers.

B. Decontaminate.

C. Airway, protect as needed.

D. O_2, high flow (10–15 L/min). Pulse oximetry will be inaccurate.

E. Utilize Cyanide Antidote Kit only with a clear indication and patient with *significant* symptoms (unconscious, confused, combative). In patient with significant symptoms:

   1. Administer amyl nitrite by inhalation. Crush ampule in handkerchief and hold in front of patient's mouth for 30 seconds, alternate with high flow oxygen every 30 seconds until IV established. Use fresh ampule every 3–4 minutes. Discontinue as soon as IV access established.

   2. IV – volume expander (NS or RL), TKO or as directed.

   3. Administer sodium nitrite 300 mg (10 ml of 3% solution) slowly IV. Rate should not exceed 2.0 ml/min. Administration by drip will assure the slower rate. If drip is preferred, mix sodium nitrite 300 mg in 50 ml NS. Begin administration at a slow rate and monitor blood pressure. Rate can be increased if blood pressure is adequate. (Target rate is 60 ml over 5–15

164

minutes.) Pediatric dose is 0.2 ml/kg, not to exceed 10 ml. Drip is preferred for the pediatric patient to avoid severe hypotension.

4. Administer sodium thiosulfate 12.5 gm (50 ml of 25% solution) slowly IV. Pediatric dose is 1.5 ml/kg, not to exceed 50 ml.

F. Administer naloxone 2 mg IV.

G. If cyanide ingested – consider charcoal or gastric lavage.

H. Transport as soon as possible – may benefit from hyperbaric oxygen therapy.

Special notes
A. Cyanide is commonly formed in many varied situations. Cyanide is a common ingredient used for pest control. It is used in metallurgy for extraction of gold and silver metals from their ores. It is used in chemical synthesis and the manufacture of many plastics. It is also found in the pits of many fruits as amygdalin, which is converted to cyanide only after it is metabolized by digestion. Finally, it has been increasingly recognized that cyanide is a byproduct of many fires; and may be a cause of death in fire victims and fire fighters more often than previously recognized.

B. Cyanide is absorbed rapidly through every route – oral, conjunctival, skin, or respiratory tract.

C. Cyanide binds to iron in the ferric state. Any enzymes which cycle between ferric and ferrous states, are susceptible to inactivation by cyanide. The cyanoferric complex is relatively stable and the enzyme remains trapped in this inactive form of the enzyme. Cyanide produces cellular hypoxia by inhibiting the reoxidation of cytochrome oxidase. This is a hemoprotein with iron in the ferric state. It is also the final step of oxidative phosphorylation which provides the primary source of energy to the cell. Blocking this step causes the cell to utilize anaerobic metabolism. This leads to an increase of lactic acid, decrease of ATP, and eventually to cellular, organ, and organism death.

D. The cytochrome oxidase-cyanide complex is dissociable. If the cyanide can be removed from the cytochrome oxidase before cellular or organism death, recovery may be the rule. The initial approach of the cyanide antidote kit is to produce methemoglobin. Both amyl nitrite and sodium nitrite will produce methemoglobinemia. This serves to attract cyanide from the cytochrome oxidase-cyanide complex to form cyanomethemoglobin complex. The methemoglobin may bind with any cyanide in the plasma, but is most effective in serving as a competitive binding site for cyanide already bound to cytochrome oxidase. Cyanomethemoglobin has relatively low toxicity. The next step in the treatment is to administer sodium thiosulfate. Sodium thiosulfate acts as a sulfur donor and permits the cyanide released from methemoglobin to combine and produce thiocyanate. The thiocyanate is relatively nontoxic and is excreted by the kidneys.

E. Many other antidotes are currently being investigated and may be available soon. Hydroxocobalamin binds cyanide without producing methemoglobin, and does not have the side effect of significant hypotension. It is currently available in some European countries, but not in the U.S.

METHEMOGLOBINEMIA

Source

A. Nitrites and nitrates

1. Sodium nitrites

2. Bismuth subnitrate (Pepto-Bismol)

3. Nitroglycerin

4. Nitroprusside (Nipride)

5. Nitrate-rich food or water

6. Silver nitrate

7. Volatile nitrites

    a. Amyl nitriteb.

    b. Butyl nitrite

    c. Isobutyl nitrite ("Rush")

B. Local anesthetics

1. Benzocaine (Unguentine, Solarcaine)

2. Lidocaine (Xylocaine)

3. Procaine (Novocain)

C. Aromatic amino and nitroso compounds

1. Aniline dyes (inks and shoe polishes)

2. Nitrobenzene

3. Phenylhydroxylamine

4. Phenazopyridine (Pyridium)

D. Miscellaneous

1. Sulfonamides (Dapsone)

2. Chlorates

3. Phenacetin

4. Primaquine

5. Methylene blue (large doses)

Clinical presentation

Methemoglobin level	Signs & Symptoms
< 10%	None
10–15%	Cyanosis
20–40%	"Chocolate cyanosis" Headache, fatigue Weakness, dizziness
40–60%	Lethargy, dyspnea Bradycardia Respiratory depression Stupor
60–80%	Seizures, coma Cardiopulmonary arrest

Treatment

A. Decontamination:

    1. Clothing removed, copious washing if external or

    2. Gastric lavage or charcoal if ingested.

B. Airway – protect as needed.

C. O_2, high flow (10–15 L/min). Pulse oximetry inaccurate.

D. IV – volume expander (NS or RL), TKO or as directed.

E. If patient severely confused, combative, or comatose:

    1. Administer naloxone 2 mg IV.

    2. Administer methylene blue 1–2 mg/kg of 1% sterile solution (10 mg/ml) slowly IV. This is equivalent to 0.1–0.2 ml/kg or total 5 to 20 ml over 10 minutes.

    3. Test blood for glucose level

    4. Administer dextrose 50%, 50 ml, IV if glucose level < 60 mg/dl.

F. Transport as soon as possible.

Special notes

A. Nitrates and nitrites have variable rates of effect depending on the route of administration. Inhalation of the volatile nitrates cause a fall in systolic blood pressure within 30 to 60 seconds with maximum effect in 1–3 minutes. The necessary metabolism of the nitrates to the methemoglobin producing nitrites would delay the onset of symptoms. Nitrates and nitrites both produce relaxation of smooth muscle in blood vessels, GI tract, bronchi, and ureters. This dilatation has long been utilized to treat patients with coronary artery disease (initially with amyl nitrites, now with nitroglycerin). At the higher doses, and with prolonged administration, however, methemoglobinemia can be a problem even from therapeutic administration of these medications.

B. Methemoglobin is an abnormal hemoglobin in which the usual reduced ferrous (Fe^{++}) state of the heme molecule is oxidized to the ferric (Fe^{+++}) form. Methemoglobin cannot reversibly bind or carry oxygen or carbon dioxide. The normal physiologic level of methemoglobin is less than 1%. Methemoglobinemia is defined as a methemoglobin level greater than 1%. Levels of 2–3% have been reported from use of amyl nitrites for 5 minutes. Intravenous nitroglycerin has been reported to produce levels over 12% on occasion. The administration of sodium nitrite 600 mg IV to treat cyanide poisoning, was reported to result in a methemoglobin level of 58% in one patient. Yet for all of the exposures, very few patients require treatment for methemoglobinemia, so many factors are involved in the metabolism and physiologic response.

C. The initial presentation of methemoglobinemia is darkened blood and a "slate gray" or "chocolate brown" cyanosis. This may be apparent only around the lips and mucous membranes. This color is the result of the pigment from the abnormal hemoglobin *not* from hypoxic cyanosis. In most normal individuals the methemoglobin level must be above 10% before the color can be distinguished.

D. Methylene blue acts as a cofactor in a reaction to accelerate the NADPH-dependent methemoglobin reductase system. This system requires the production of reduced NADPH by the pentose phosphate shunt, the reductase enzyme and cofactor such as methylene blue. The result is the reduced (functional) form of hemoglobin being produced from the methemoglobin (nonfunctional) form.

SULFIDES

A. Hydrogen sulfide

B. Carbon disulfide

C. Mercaptans

D. Sulfides found or used in

   1. Sulfur springs
   6. Petroleum industry

   2. Volcanic gases
   7. Farming

   3. Liquid manure
   8. Jet fuels

   4. Insecticides
   9. Metal refining

   5. Soil fumigants

E. Sulfides used in the manufacturing of

   1. Rubber
   4. Leather

   2. Synthetic fabrics
   5. Plastics

   3. Heavy water
   6. Asphalt

Clinical presentation

A. Low concentration

   1. Irritation
     Eye – "gas eye", keratoconjunctivitis
     Respiratory tract (pharyngitis, bronchitis)
     Gastrointestinal tract

   2. Headache

   3. Nausea and vomiting

   4. Weakness

B. High concentration

   1. Neurologic – Agitation, seizures, coma, respiratory paralysis.

   2. Cardiac – Disorders of conduction, various dysrhythmias.

   3. Local – Caustic burn.

Treatment

A. Assure safety of rescuers.

B. Decontaminate.

C. Airway, protect as needed.

D. O_2, high flow (10–15 L/min). Pulse oximetry will be inaccurate.

E. Administer amyl nitrite by inhalation. Crush ampule in handkerchief and hold in front of patient's mouth for 30 seconds, alternate with high flow oxygen every 30 second until IV established.

F. IV – Volume expander (NS or RL), TKO or as directed.

G. Administer sodium nitrite 300 mg (10 ml or 3% solution) slowly IV. Rate should not exceed 2.0 ml/min. Pediatric dose is 0.2 ml/kg, not to exceed 10 ml. Administer *very slowly* or as drip.

H. Observe for seizures and treat with diazepam 5–10 mg IV slowly until seizure stops or 10 mg has been given.

I. Observe for signs of acute pulmonary edema and treat as necessary

J. Transport as soon as possible – may benefit from hyperbaric oxygen therapy.

Special notes

A. Hydrogen sulfide is absorbed primarily through inhalation. Percutaneous absorption is minimal, although toxicity has been reported following application of sulfur-containing dermatologic preparations. Hydrogen sulfide is a highly toxic, odorous ("rotten egg" smell), and irritating gas. It is the cause of a number of fatalities, many multiple, due to inadequately protected rescuers.

B. Hydrogen sulfide, like cyanide, binds to cytochrome oxidase and prevents aerobic metabolism at the cellular level. The administration of sodium nitrite induces methemoglobinemia which acts as a competitor with cytochrome oxidase to draw the sulfide off the enzyme to form sulfmethemoglobin. This is a relatively benign compound that is auto degraded to nontoxic forms of sulfur, which are excreted by the kidneys.

FLUORIDE

Source
A. Hydrofluoric acid

    1. Glass etching

    2. Petroleum refining

    3. Dental work

    4. Rust removal

    5. Fertilizers

    6. Manufacturing

      a. Fire extinguishers

      b. Dyes

      c. Tanning agents

      d. Refrigerants

      e. Plastics

B. Other fluoride compounds

    1. Sodium fluoride

    2. Cryolite

    3. Toothpaste, mouthwashes

    4. Insecticides and rodenticides

    5. Dietary supplements

Clinical presentation

Skin – Concentrated hydrofluoric acid causes lesions which are immediately, intensely painful. Dilute acid can delay treatment with prolonged absorption.

Lungs – Concentrated vapors are intensely irritating to lungs and conjunctivae. May lead to respiratory tract damage and pulmonary edema.

GI – Direct corrosive effect – nausea, vomiting and abdominal pain.

Other:

A. Fluoride ion chelates calcium – lower serum calcium may result in paresthesias, tetany, convulsions and cardiac dysrhythmias.

B. Fluoride impairs the formation of collagen tissue and has direct action on muscle and nerve tissue. May result in a variety of musculoskeletal and neurologic complaints, including headache, paresthesias, visual disturbances, and mental deterioration.

C. Fluoride interferes with many enzyme systems – glycolytic enzymes, cholinesterases, and others.

Treatment

A. Assure safety of rescuers.

B. Decontaminate.

C. Airway, protect as needed.

D. O_2, high flow (10–15 L/min). Titrate to pulse oximetry > 90% if possible.

E. IV – volume expander (NS or RL), wide open to 20 ml/kg, unless contraindicated by pulmonary edema.

F. Cardiac monitor.

G. Apply calcium gluconate gel to any skin lesions which are symptomatic.

H. For patients with significant exposure and signs of hypocalcemia – administer calcium gluconate, 10% solution 5–10 ml slowly IV. Pediatric dose 0.2 ml/kg.

I. Consider administration of magnesium sulfate 1–2 gm IV.

J. Transport as soon as possible.

Special notes

A. Hydrofluoric acid is one of the strongest acids known. It is used extensively in chemical and industrial plants for a variety of applications. On direct contact hydrofluoric acid causes liquefaction necrosis by action of the hydrogen ion that is identical to other acid burns, disrupting the outer layer of skin and immediately proceeding to destroy the subcutaneous tissues. The fluoride ion penetrates into the subcutaneous tissues and complexes with calcium and magnesium to form insoluble fluoride salts. This process continues and can result in hypocalcemia or hypomagnesemia.

B. The fluoride ion also acts as an enzyme inhibitor which inhibits cellular metabolism. Severe hydrofluoric acid burns can be associated with systemic fluoride toxicity.

7

PREHOSPITAL PROCEDURES: BASIC AND ADVANCED

INTRODUCTION

Prehospital procedures, both basic and advanced, are listed in alphabetical order. Basic procedures are appropriate to basic EMTs as well as to Paramedic level personnel:

Airway management: Opening airway
Obstructed airway
Clearing and suctioning
Assisting ventilation

Bandaging
Defibrillation (AED)
PASG application
Splinting, extremity
Splinting, spine

Advanced procedures are those techniques which require physician direction in teaching, skill maintenance, and use. Some procedures are suitable for standing-order by agreement:

Airway management: Orotracheal intubation
Nasotracheal intubation
Dual lumen airways

Airway monitoring: Pulse oximetry and Capnography
Defibrillation
Intraosseous cannulation
Medication administration
Peripheral IV insertion

Others are controversial and require regional consensus before use. By including these procedures, we do not intend to endorse their use by all personnel. Each has been found useful on some occasion within our system; but all have low frequency of use, and a sometimes unacceptably high risk of patient injury. They should be performed only by *direct physician order* at the time of the occurrence whenever possible.

Cardioversion
Carotid sinus massage
Cricothyrotomy
Foley catheter insertion (long transports only)
ICD magnet
NG tube insertion (long transports only)
Tension pneumothorax decompression

AIRWAY MANAGEMENT

General Principles

The numerous airway procedures which follow are insufficient in themselves, unless the EMT or Paramedic can decide in a practical situation which form of management should be used. The following principles should be remembered in the "heat of battle" to allow optimum care of the airway without unnecessary intervention.

1. Use the simplest method of airway management appropriate to the patient.

2. Use the method with which the emergency responder is most comfortable.

3. Use meticulous suctioning to keep the airway clear of debris.

4. Monitor continuously to be sure that the treatment is still effective.

5. Understand the difference between various aspects of the airway management.

   a. Patency – how open and clear is the airway, free of foreign substances, blood, vomitus and tongue.

   b. Ventilation – the amount of air the patient is able to inhale and exhale in a given time.

   c. Oxygenation – the amount of oxygen the patient is carrying to his tissues.

Each needs to be treated separately and requires different techniques and equipment.

The following protocols are recommended as a guide for approaching difficult medical and trauma airway problems. They assume that the responder is skilled in the various procedures and the protocols will need to be modified according to training level. Advanced procedures should only be attempted if simpler ones fail and if the technician is qualified. Individual cases may require modification of these protocols.

Medical Respiratory Arrest

1. Open airway using head-tilt/chin-lift or jaw-thrust maneuver.

2. Look, listen and feel for spontaneous respirations.

3. Apply pocket mask (or BVM) with supplemental oxygen to ventilate.

4. Insert nasopharyngeal airway or oropharyngeal airway if patency difficult to maintain.

5. Suction as needed.

6. Perform orotracheal intubation after patient otherwise stabilized prior to transport if arrest continues.

Medical Respiratory Insufficiency

1. Open the airway using most efficient method.

2. Insert nasopharyngeal airway.

3. Suction as needed.

4 Apply supplemental O_2 by nasal cannula or mask as needed.

5. Assist respirations by pocket mask or bag-valve-mask as needed.

6. Perform nasotracheal or orotracheal intubation if prolonged support is needed, or if airway requires continued protection from aspiration.

Traumatic Respiratory Arrest

1. Open airway using jaw-thrust maneuver, protecting neck.

2. Clear the airway using finger sweep, suction as needed.

3. Have assistant stabilize head and neck.

4. Use towel clip or hand to draw tongue and mandible forward if needed in patients with facial injuries.

5. Use pocket mask or bag-valve-mask for initial control of ventilation.

6. Perform orotracheal intubation with neck stabilized. Pressure over larynx may make intubation easier.

7. If intubation cannot be performed due to severe facial injury, *and* patient cannot be ventilated with mask – *perform cricothyroid stick or cricothyrotomy. Cricothyrotomy is a difficult and hazardous technique which should only be used in extraordinary circumstances.

Traumatic Respiratory Insufficiency

1. Open airway using jaw-thrust maneuver, protecting neck.

2. Clear the airway using finger sweep. Suction as needed.

3. Have assistant provide continuous stabilization to head and neck.

4. Use towel clip or hand to draw tongue and mandible forward if needed with facial injuries.

5. Supplement with O_2, support with mask ventilation.

6. Attempt nasotracheal intubation to secure airway if needed and if no significant midface trauma.

7. If patient deteriorates and cannot be supported by less invasive means:

   a. Attempt orotracheal intubation with neck stabilized.

   b. *Perform cricothyroid stick or cricothyrotomy and use high frequency jet ventilation if available. Cricothyrotomy is a difficult and hazardous technique which should only be used in extraordinary circumstances.

Although cricothyroid stick and cricothyrotomy are hazardous procedures and have been listed as DIRECT PHYSICIAN ORDER procedures, it is apparent that in circumstances where these techniques are actually essential for the patient's airway – there may be no time to make a phone/radio call. In those "time critical" instances, it is better to perform the needed procedure, then document the circumstances in an incident report.

Discussion

Stepwise procedures for obtaining control of the airway in medical situations have been well accepted and standardized by AHA protocol as well as practical clinical experience. We would encourage more widespread use of nasopharyngeal airways in lightly comatose patients who still require some support for a lax tongue. Nasotracheal intubation is another alternative in breathing patients who require intervention.

But when is active control of the airway needed? In many instances, the maximally invasive form of airway management is chosen because of incorrect judgments about "impending" respiratory arrest.

Especially with head injuries, it is hard to predict. An irregular breathing pattern may represent chaotic breathing rather than impending arrest. On the other hand, despite the obvious risks of active airway management, the risks of inadequate oxygenation are even greater. Both under treatment and over treatment may be costly to the patient. It is better to err on the side of aggressive airway management when necessary to achieve adequate oxygenation.

The unsolved problem of emergency airway management is what to do with the patient who requires active airway management and has a potential cervical spine injury. Clearly no one wishes to save a life at the expense of producing a quadriplegic. Nevertheless, if the patient is not breathing adequately to what avail is it to save the spinal cord function, if the patient is vegetated or dies because of prolonged attempts to perform difficult operative procedures with inadequate experience. Currently, the best method to control the airway is to intubate orally with an assistant maintaining stabilization (digital intubation, also with stabilization, is an alternative). In a non-arrested patient, nasotracheal intubation is an alternative if there is no midface trauma. Multiple dual lumen airway devices have recently been developed. They may provide a reasonable alternative in the patient who is impossible to intubate. Technical competence requires good training, adequate practice, and compulsive attention to detail to ensure safe and effective performance of any procedure. Cricothyrotomy remains the only alternative for a small number of patients who have injuries that preclude routine airway procedures.

AIRWAY MANAGEMENT: OPENING THE AIRWAY

Indications
A. Inadequate air exchange in the lungs due to jaw or facial fracture causing narrowing of air passage.

B. Lax jaw or tongue muscles causing airway narrowing in the unconscious patient.

C. Noisy breathing or excessive respiratory effort due to partial obstruction.

D. In preparation for suctioning, assisted ventilation or other airway management maneuvers.

Precautions
Wear gloves and eye protection.

A. For trauma victims, keep neck in midline and avoid flexion or hyperextension.

B. For medical patients, neck extension may be difficult in elderly persons with extensive arthritis and little neck motion. Do not use force. Jaw-thrust or chin-lift without head-tilt will be more successful.

C. All airway maneuvers should be followed by an evaluation of their success. If breathing is still labored, a different method or more time for recovery may be needed.

D. Children's airways have less supporting cartilage. Overextension can kink the airway and increase the obstruction. Watch chest movement to determine the best head angle.

E. Dentures should usually be left in place since they provide a framework for the lips and cheeks and allow a more effective seal for ventilation.

Technique
A. To *open the airway* initially, choose method most suitable for patient – See Table 7-1. Assess ventilation (Figure 7-1).

B. Begin ventilation with bag-valve-mask if patient is not breathing.

C. Relieve partial or complete obstruction, if present.

181

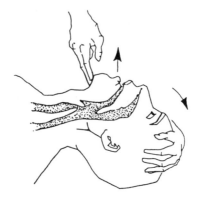

Figure 7-1. Opening Airway

D. Assess oxygenation. Use supplemental O_2 as needed.

E. Choose method to *maintain airway patency* during transport:

    1. Position patient on side (if medical problem).

    2. Oropharyngeal airway (Figure 7-2):

        a. Choose size by measuring from mouth to margin of ear.

        b. Depress tongue with tongue blade, or insert gently with the curve pointing *upward*. Avoid snagging posterior tongue or palate.

        c. Insert to back of tongue, then turn to follow curve of airway. Move gently to be sure the tip is free in back of pharynx.

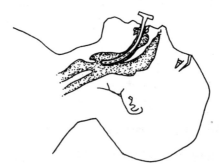

Figure 7-2. Oropharyngeal Airway

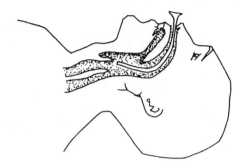

Figure 7-3. Nasopharyngeal Airway

3. Nasopharyngeal airway (Figure 7-3):

   a. Lubricate tube gently.

   b. Insert in right nostril, along floor of nose until flange is seated at the nostril. Keep curve in line with normal airway curve. If you meet resistance, try the left side.

F. Listen to breathing to be sure maneuver has resolved problem.

G. Consider intubation to provide adequate airway.

H. Resume ventilatory assistance and oxygenation as appropriate.

I. Consider cricothyrotomy *only* if unable to intubate. Cricothyrotomy is a difficult and hazardous technique which should be used only in extraordinary circumstances.

Complications

A. Cervical spinal cord injury from neck hyperextension in trauma victim with cervical fracture.

B. Neck fracture in older patients with rigid neck due to forced extension during airway maneuvers.

C. Death due to inadequate ventilation or hypoxia.

D. Nasal or posterior pharyngeal bleeding due to trauma from tubes.

E. Increased airway obstruction from tongue following improper oropharyngeal airway placement.

F. Aspiration of blood or vomitus from inadequate suctioning and continued contamination of lungs from upper airway.

Special Notes

A. Researchers have found that the head-tilt/chin-lift is successful at least as often as the head-tilt/neck-lift and that it may be more reliable and less fatiguing. Unfortunately, it cannot be simulated on mannikins, but with use, it is easy to get comfortable with this technique.

B. During transport, medical patients can be placed in a *stable position* on their sides for effective airway control. Use a flexed leg, arm, or pillow for support. Our supine "packaging" of patients for transport is often the worst way to ensure an adequate airway.

C. Nasopharyngeal airways are very useful for airway maintenance. The nasal insertion provides more stability, the airway is better tolerated in partially awake patients, and it does not carry the risk of blocking the airway further like the stiff oropharyngeal airway.

TABLE 7-1.   METHODS OF OPENING THE AIRWAY

Head-tilt/chin-lift

Technique – From beside head, place one hand on forehead. Grasp lower edge of chin with fingers of other hand and lift chin forward (Figure 7-1). Teeth may come together.

Indications – Medical patient. May require less neck extension than head tilt. Useful with dentures. May be used without head-tilt in trauma victims.

Jaw thrust

Technique – Position yourself above patient. Place fingers of each hand under angle of jaw, just below ears. Lift jaw, using forearms to maintain head alignment (Figure 7-4).

Indications – Trauma victim or medical patient where neck extension is not possible. Bag-valve-mask ventilation must be done by another rescuer and this is a fatiguing method. May be used with dentures in place.

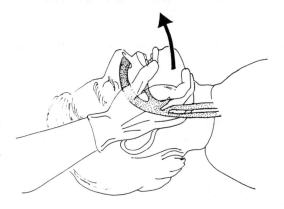

Figure 7-4. Jaw thrust

AIRWAY MANAGEMENT: OBSTRUCTED AIRWAY

Indications

A. Complete or partial obstruction of the airway due to a foreign body.

B. Complete or partial obstruction due to airway swelling from anaphylaxis, croup, or epiglottitis.

C. Patient with unknown illness or injury who cannot be ventilated after opening the airway.

Precautions

Wear gloves and eye protection.

A. Perform *chest thrusts only* in patients who are visibly pregnant, obese, or infants.

B. Patients with partial airway obstruction can be very uncomfortable and vociferous. Abdominal or chest thrusts will not be effective and may be injurious to the patient who is still ventilating. Resist the temptation to attempt relief of obstruction if it is not complete, but be ready to intervene promptly if arrest occurs.

C. Hypoxia from airway obstruction can cause seizures. Chest or abdominal thrusts may not be effective until the patient becomes relaxed after the seizure is over.

Technique

Complete airway obstruction

A. Open airway using head-tilt/chin-lift.

B. Attempt to ventilate.

C. If unable to ventilate, reposition airway and re-attempt ventilation.

D. If airway remains obstructed, visualize with laryngoscope and remove any obvious foreign body.

E. Reposition the airway and attempt to ventilate.

F. If unable to ventilate, administer up to five (5) subdiaphragmatic abdominal thrusts.

G. Reposition the airway and reattempt to ventilate.

H. *Consider cricothyrotomy if obstruction unrelieved.

I. When obstruction relieved:

1. Keep patient on side, sweep airway to remove debris.

2. Apply O_2, high flow (10–15 L/min) by mask. Titrate to pulse oximetry > 90% if possible.

3. Assess adequacy of ventilation and support as needed.

4. Suction aggressively.

5. Gently restrain if combative or confused.

Partial airway obstruction
A. Have patient assume most comfortable position.

B. Apply O_2, high flow (10–15 L/min) by mask or as high as possible through nasal cannula if mask would hinder efforts to assist patient. Titrate pulse oximetry to 90% if possible.

C. Attempt suctioning of upper airway *if* patient can lie on side to protect airway and cooperate with suctioning.

D. If patient unable to move air, confused, or otherwise deteriorating – visualize airway, remove foreign body or perform abdominal thrusts as noted above.

Complications
A. Hypoxic brain damage and death from unrecognized or unrelieved obstruction.

B. Trauma to ribs, lung, liver and spleen from chest or abdominal thrusts (particularly when forces not evenly distributed).

C. Vomiting and aspiration after relief of obstruction.

D. Creation of complete obstruction after incorrect finger probing.

E. Tonsillar or pharyngeal laceration from over-vigorous finger sweep.

Special Notes
A. Occasionally, patients will have a better airway in the supine than in the upright position. Let the patient assume his position of comfort.

187

B. Be prepared! Patients who are relieved of airway obstruction usually vomit. They may also be confused enough after the hypoxic episode that they are unable to clear their secretions. There is no substitute for careful and aggressive suctioning.

C. Technique of proper abdominal and chest thrusts as well as airway positions and sweeps is found in basic CPR texts. Persons who have relieved obstruction say that after 1 or 2 thrusts, it becomes very clear how much force will be needed to "pop the cork". Prehospital providers should be meticulous in their technique to minimize the possibility of injury to patient and maximize likelihood of success.

AIRWAY MANAGEMENT: CLEARING AND SUCTIONING THE AIRWAY

Indications
A. Trauma to the upper airway, with blood, teeth, or other material causing partial obstruction.

B. Vomitus, food boluses or foreign material in airway.

C. Excess secretions or pulmonary edema fluid in upper airway or lungs (with endotracheal tube in place).

D. Meconium or amniotic fluid in mouth, nose and oropharynx of newborn.

Precautions
Wear gloves and eye protection.

A. Suctioning, particularly through endotracheal tubes, always risks suctioning the available oxygen, as well as the fluid, from the airway. Limit the suction time to a few seconds while the catheter is being withdrawn.

B. This precaution should *not* be followed when vomitus or other material continues to well up and completely obstruct airway. In those situations suctioning must be continued until an airway is re-established.

C. Use equipment large enough for the job at hand. Pepperoni will not be cleared out with hard tonsil suckers. Large amount of particulate matter requires open-ended suction with connecting tubing.

D. The catheter and tubing will require frequent rinsing with water or saline to permit continued suctioning. Have a bottle of water or saline at hand before you begin, Use gauze to remove large material from the end of the catheter.

E. Never attempt to *insert* a suction catheter with the suction functioning. Suction only on *withdrawal* of the catheter.

Technique
A. Open airway and inspect for visible foreign material.

B. Turn patient on side if possible to facilitate clearance.

189

C. Remove large or obvious foreign matter with gloved hands. Use padded tongue blade or oropharyngeal airway (do not pry) to keep airway open. Sweep finger *across* posterior pharynx and clear material out of mouth.

D. Attach suction machine and test motor.

E. *Suction* of oropharynx (Figure 7-5)

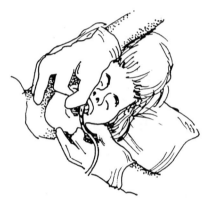

Figure 7-5. Suctioning

1. Attach tonsil tip (or use open end for large amount of debris).

2. Ventilate and oxygenate the patient prior to the procedure as needed.

3. Insert tip into oropharynx under direct vision with sweeping motion.

4. Pinch tubing or block suction while advancing to posterior pharynx.

5. Suction as the tip is gently withdrawn back through mouth.

6. Continue intermittent suction interspersed with active oxygenation by mask or cannula. Use positive pressure ventilation if needed.

7. If suction becomes clogged, dilute by suctioning water from a glass to unclog tubing. If suction clogs repeatedly, use connecting tubing alone or manually remove large debris.

F. *Catheter suction* of endotracheal tube

1. Attach suction catheter to tubing of suction device (leaving suction end in sterile container).

2. Hyperventilate patient 4–5 times rapidly.

3. Put on sterile gloves if possible.

4. Detach bag from endotracheal tube and insert sterile tip of suction catheter *without* suction.

5. When catheter tip has been *gently* advanced as far as possible, apply suction and withdraw catheter slowly.

6. Rinse catheter tip in sterile water or saline.

7. Hyperventilate patient before each suction attempt.

G. *Bulb suction* of newborn

1. As soon as infant's head has delivered, insert suction tip (with bulb compressed) into the nose – then release bulb while withdrawing from nose.

2. Suction each nostril, then mouth if time allows.

3. As soon as infant has delivered, repeat process, suctioning first the mouth then the nostrils.

4. Suction trachea under direct vision with laryngoscope if there is evidence of meconium aspiration.

Complications

A. Hypoxia due to excessive suctioning time without adequate ventilation between attempts.

B. Persistent obstruction due to inadequate tubing size for removal of debris.

C. Lung injury from aspiration of stomach contents due to inadequate suctioning.

D. Asphyxia due to recurrent obstruction if airway is not monitored after initial suctioning.

E. Conversion of partial to complete obstruction by attempts at airway clearance.

F. Trauma to the posterior pharynx from forced use of equipment.

G. Vomiting and aspiration from stimulation of gag reflex.

H. Induction of cardiorespiratory arrest from vagal stimulation.

Special Notes

A. Bulb suction can be used on the newborn but is not as effective as direct visualization and suction, particularly if there is any meconium to aspirate.

B. Patients with pulmonary edema may have endless frothy secretions. Be sure to allow time for the patient to breathe, even though it is tempting to continue suctioning.

C. Vomiting by rescuer can occur when managing patients with airway obstruction from food and vomitus. Resume treatment as soon as possible.

D. Complications may be caused both by inadequate and overly vigorous suctioning. Technique and choice of equipment are very important. Choose equipment with enough power to suction large amounts rapidly to allow time for ventilation.

E. Proper airway clearance can make the difference between a patient who survives and one who dies. Airway obstruction is one of the most common treatable causes of prehospital death.

AIRWAY MANAGEMENT: ASSISTING VENTILATION

Indications
A. Inadequate patient ventilation due to fatigue, coma, or other causes for respiratory depression.

B. To apply positive pressure breathing in patients with pulmonary edema and severe fatigue.

C. To ventilate patients in respiratory arrest.

D. For use in conjunction with ET tube to ventilate. (BVM or demand valve can be used for this purpose.)

Precautions
Wear gloves and eye protection.

A. Mouth-to-mouth ventilation in the field should seldom be necessary for a professional response team. Airway equipment should always be readily available.

B. However, if mouth-to-mouth has been used, it is unlikely any diseases would be passed to the rescuer during the time of ventilatory assistance. Check with the doctor at the receiving hospital if you have any particular concerns. Pocket masks are particularly useful for rapid airway assistance.

C. Oxygen-powered breathing devices are very easy to use, but potentially most dangerous. You cannot feel the patient resistance and airway patency. The loud hiss can be impressive but still just ventilate the surrounding atmosphere. Watch chest movement carefully!

D. Bag-valve-mask (BVM) devices were developed for use in a controlled operating room setting. Ventilation in a field situation can be much less satisfactory. Two people are often required to obtain an adequate mask fit and also ventilate. Pocket masks can be much easier and more effective in some circumstances.

Technique
A. Open the airway.

B. Check for ventilation.

C. If patient is not breathing, perform 2 full breaths and check pulse. Begin CPR as needed.

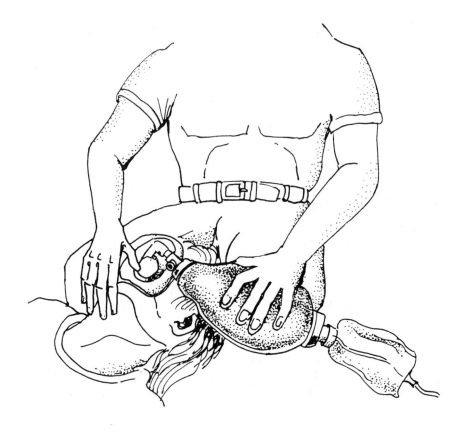

Figure 7-6. Bag-valve-mask ventilation

D. If pulse is present but patient is not breathing, continue pocket mask ventilation until adjuncts are available.

E. Attach O_2 to pocket mask or BVM.

F. Position yourself above patient's head, continue to hold airway position, seat mask firmly on the face, and begin assisted ventilation (Figure 7-6).

G. Watch chest for rise and feel for air leak or resistance to air passage. Adjust mask fit as needed.

H. If patient resumes spontaneous respirations, attach mask strap and continue to administer supplemental oxygen. Intermittent assistance with ventilation may still be needed.

I. If demand valve is to be used, again position yourself above patient, get secure mask fit. Depress button and observe for chest rise (1–2 seconds). Release and allow patient to exhale. (Exhalation should be longer than inhalation for most patients.) *Be sure airway is open to avoid gastric distention. Also, avoid hyperinflation.*

Complications

A. Continued aspiration of blood, vomitus, and other upper airway debris.

B. Inadequate ventilation due to poor seal between patient's mouth and ventilatory device.

C. Gastric distention, possibly causing vomiting. This can be particularly severe with demand valve use.

D. Trauma to the upper airway from forcible use of airways.

E. With demand valves – pneumothorax development or other lung injury from high pressure ventilation.

F. Pneumothorax in children.

Special Notes

A. Basic airway management will be less than adequate over long distances in the patient who continues to bleed or vomit into his upper airway. This patient will benefit from the advanced airway management techniques involved in nasotracheal or orotracheal intubation.

B. For children, flip the pocket mask so the narrow end is toward the chin and cover both nose and mouth while ventilating.

C. Assisted ventilation will not hurt a patient and should be used whenever the breathing pattern seems shallow, slow, or otherwise abnormal. Do not be afraid to be aggressive about assisting ventilation, even in patients who do not require or will not tolerate intubation. (If the patient is awake enough to resist, he is probably OK without help.)

ADVANCED AIRWAY MANAGEMENT: OROTRACHEAL INTUBATION

Indications

In most cases, orotracheal intubation provides definitive control of the airway. Its purposes include:

A. Active ventilation of the patient.

B. Delivery of high concentrations of oxygen.

C. Suctioning secretions and maintaining airway patency.

D. Prevention of aspiration (gastric contents, upper airway secretions, or bleeding).

E. Prevention of gastric distention due to assisted ventilation.

F. Administration of positive pressure when extra fluid is present in alveoli.

G. Administration of drugs during resuscitation for absorption through the lungs.

H. Allowing more effective CPR.

I. Allowing hyperventilation to decrease PCO_2, and thus, decrease intracranial pressure.

Precautions

Wear gloves and eye protection.

A. Do not use intubation as the primary method of managing the airway in an arrest. Oxygenation prior to intubation should be accomplished with mouth-to-mask or bag-valve-mask, as needed.

B. Neck movement should be avoided in the trauma patient. Oral intubation with cervical stabilization is usually the best choice for a trauma patient requiring definitive airway control. Nasotracheal intubation is a good alternative in the breathing patient with no mid-face trauma.

C. Never lever the laryngoscope against the teeth. The jaw should be lifted with direct upward traction by the laryngoscope.

D. Prepare suction beforehand. Vomiting is particularly common when the esophagus is intubated.

E. Intubation should take no more than 15–20 seconds to complete. Do not lose track of time. If the visualization is difficult, stop and reventilate before trying again.

Technique

A. Assemble the equipment while continuing ventilation:

   1. Choose tube size (see Table 7.2 below).

   2. Introduce the stylette and be sure it stops ½" short of the tube's end.

   3. Assemble laryngoscope and check light.

   4. Connect and check suction.

B. Position patient – neck flexed forward, head extended back. Back of head should be level with or higher than back of shoulders.

C. Give a minimum of 4 good ventilations before starting procedure.

D. Insert laryngoscope to right of midline. Move it to midline, pushing tongue to left and out of view.

E. Lift straight up on blade (no levering) to expose posterior pharynx.

F. Identify epiglottis – tip of *curved blade* should sit in vallecula (Figure 7-7) (in front of epiglottis), *straight blade* should slip over epiglottis (Figure 7-8).

G. With gentle further traction to straighten the airway, identify trachea from arytenoid cartilages and vocal cords (Figure 7-9).

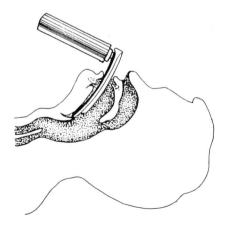
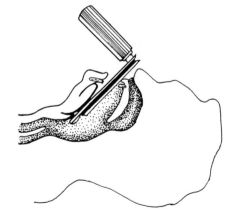

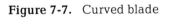

Figure 7-7. Curved blade   **Figure 7-8.** Straight blade

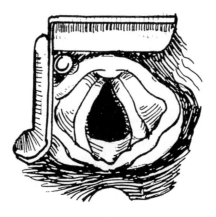

Figure 7-9. Vocal cords

H. Insert tube from right side of mouth, along blade, into trachea under *direct vision*.

I. Advance tube so cuff is 1–1.5" beyond cords. Ventilate and watch for chest rise. Listen for breath sounds over stomach (should not be heard) and lungs and axillae.

J. Inflate cuff with 5–10 ml air (balloon should be full, but not hard), clamp if necessary to secure against leaks.

K. Re-auscultate over stomach and both sides of chest.

L. In patient with signs of life (pulse or respiratory effort) measure expired CO_2, if possible.

M. Note proper tube position and secure tube with tape if adequate expired CO_2.

Complications

A. Esophageal intubation – particularly common when tube not visualized as it passes through cords. The greatest danger is in not recognizing the error. Auscultation over stomach during trial ventilation should reveal air gurgling through gastric contents with esophageal placement. Also, make sure patient's color improves as it should when ventilating. Expired CO_2 measurement will help prevent this complication as well as the suction device which will suction air freely from the trachea, but is unable to suction from the esophagus which immediately collapses around the tube.

B. Intubation of right mainstem bronchus – listen to the chest bilaterally.

C. Upper airway trauma due to excess force with laryngoscope or to traumatic tube placement.

D. Vomiting and aspiration during traumatic intubation or intubation of patient with intact gag reflex.

E. Hypoxia due to prolonged intubation attempt.

F. Cervical spine fracture or cord damage in patients with arthritis and poor cervical mobility.

G. Cervical cord damage in trauma victims with spine injury.

H. Ventricular dysrhythmias or fibrillation in hypothermia patients from stimulation of airway.

I. Induction of pneumothorax, either from traumatic insertion, forceful bagging, or aggravation of underlying pneumothorax.

Special Notes
A. Orotracheal intubation can be accomplished in trauma victims if an assistant maintains stabilization and keeps the neck in neutral position. Careful visualization with the laryngoscope is needed and McGill forceps may be helpful in guiding the ET tube.

B. *Remember:* Endotracheal intubation is *not* the procedure of choice in the first minutes of a resuscitation. It is a secondary procedure only. Most persons can be adequately ventilated with pocket mask or BVM with oropharyngeal or nasopharyngeal airway. Wait to intubate until the situation is under enough control that the procedure will be successful.

C. Difficult intubations can occasionally be made easier by continuous pressure placed over the thyroid and cricoid cartilages, moving the vocal cords posteriorly into view.

D. Do not be overly aggressive and quick to intubate in trauma victims with upper airway trauma. If you are able to manage secretions and ventilate, intubation is often not required and the complications may outweigh the advantages if your hand is not forced.

E. Increased intracranial pressure frequently will result from attempts at intubation. Administration of lidocaine, 1.5 mg/kg IV, one minute before intubation attempts, may decrease this risk. Do not delay intubation, however, for IV efforts in patient with no respirations.

F. End-tidal CO_2 detection is a new tool to help confirm proper tube placement in patients with intact circulatory status. Those patients, when intubated properly should have a measurable expired CO_2 level which will confirm tube placement. Patients in cardiac arrest may have no expired CO_2 because of low blood flow through the lungs, resulting in poor or no gas exchange. CO_2 measurement in these patients may add to the confusion, rather than assist the evaluation.

TABLE 7-2.   OROTRACHEAL TUBE SIZE

Age	Endotracheal Tube
Preemie	2.5–3.0 Uncuffed
Newborn	3.0–3.5
6 months	3.5
18 months	4.0
3 years	4.5
5 years	5.0
8 years	6.0 Cuffed
10–15 years	6.5–7.0 Cuffed
Adult	7.0–9.0 Cuffed

ADVANCED AIRWAY MANAGEMENT: NASOTRACHEAL INTUBATION

Indications
A. Same function as orotracheal intubation.

B. Use when intubation is indicated but when direct visualization of the posterior pharynx is contra-indicated because of difficulty with oral access or the possibility of neck injury.

C. Most useful in breathing, comatose patients requiring intubation. May be better tolerated in partly conscious patients. *Not indicated for respiratory arrest.*

D. Asthma or pulmonary edema, with respiratory failure, where intubation may need to be achieved in a sitting position.

Precautions
Wear gloves and eye protection.

A. Head must be exactly in midline for successful intubation.

B. Have suction ready. Vomiting can occur as with any stimulation of the airway. Nose bleeds are common and can further compromise the airway. Use gentle technique to decrease risk of additional problems.

C. Nasotracheal intubation is more time-consuming than orotracheal intubation. *Therefore, it is especially true that this is not an "emergent" procedure.* The patient should be ventilating and the situation should be calm enough to be able to hear the air exchange.

D. Often nares are asymmetrical and one side is much easier to intubate. Avoid inducing bilateral nasal hemorrhage by forcing a nasotracheal tube on multiple attempts.

E. Do not use in patients with significant nasal or craniofacial trauma.

Technique
A. Choose correct ET tube size (usually 7 mm tube in adult). Limitation is nasal canal diameter.

B. Position patient with head in midline, neutral position (cervical collar may be in place or assistant may provide cervical stabilization in trauma patients).

C. Administer neosynephrine nasal spray in both nostrils.

D. Assist ventilation prior to procedure if spontaneous respirations are inadequate.

E. Lubricate ET tube with Xylocaine jelly or other lubricant.

F. With gentle steady pressure, advance the tube through the nose to the posterior pharynx. Use right nostril if possible.

G. Keeping the curve of the tube exactly in midline, continue advancing slowly.

H. There will be a slight resistance just before entering trachea. Wait for an inspiratory effort before final advance into trachea. Patient may also cough or buck just before breath.

I. Continue advancing until air is exchanging through the tube.

J. Advance about one inch further, then inflate cuff.

K. Ventilate and check for breath sounds bilaterally.

L. In patient with signs of life (pulse or respiratory effort) measure expired CO_2, if possible.

M. Note proper tube position and tape securely, if adequate expired CO_2.

Complications
Same as orotracheal intubation. In addition:

A. Further craniofacial injury, particularly in patients presenting with facial trauma.

B. Upper airway bleeding caused by tube trauma.

C. Vomiting and aspiration in the patient with intact gag reflex.

Special Notes
A. Blind nasotracheal intubation is a very "elegant" technique. In the field, the secret of blind intubation is perfect positioning and gentle patience.

B. Nasotracheal intubation should be a *gentle* alternative to orotracheal intubation. It is not indicated for the struggling, combative patient who will be the most likely to develop epistaxis which can add to the airway difficulties. It is also not indicated to test for "true" responsiveness in the unconscious patient (although sometimes you may indeed learn that they were not as deeply unconscious as previously supposed.)

C. In patients without neck injury, a laryngoscope may be used to visualize the tube. McGill forceps are useful to direct it.

D. Nasotracheal tubes often must be replaced in the patient who will require ongoing intubation and pulmonary care. The orotracheal route may be preferred for the 1–2 mm increased size tube which may permit better suctioning and improved ventilation. Consider all of the alternatives when selecting an airway.

E. End-tidal CO_2 measurement should be most helpful in the patient who is intubated with a nasotracheal tube. This presupposes that the patient is having some respiratory effort with intact cardiovascular system. CO_2 measurements should reliably indicate expired CO_2 in these patients if they are properly intubated.

ADVANCED AIRWAY MANAGEMENT: DUAL LUMEN AIRWAY DEVICES

Indications

A. Inability to intubate patient who is in need of airway protection.

B. Difficulty with intubation when rapid control of the airway is essential.

C. Primary means of airway control for personnel trained in the use of these devices only. Requires regional consensus for use.

D. May be particularly useful for patients with facial or cervical spine abnormalities.

Precautions

Wear gloves and eye protection.

A. Current devices are not indicated or appropriate for pediatric patients. (Not for use under 5' tall or younger than 16.)

B. Cannot be used in patients with intact gag reflex.

C. Should not be used in patients who have ingested caustic substances.

D. Should not be used in patients with known esophageal disease.

E. Should be used with caution in patients who have broken teeth or dental work that may tear the balloons. Insert cautiously, and try to avoid the sharp edges.

Technique

A. Initiate airway control with primary methods: CPR, mouth-to-mask, or bag-valve-mask with oxygen.

B. Assemble equipment and check balloons. Lubricate distal tip with water soluble lubricant if necessary. Assure a slight bend in the tube to conform with the airway.

C. Suction upper airway if needed.

D. In trauma patients, have assistant maintain neutral alignment of head and neck, avoiding hyperextension. In medical patients, simply position head in neutral position, hyperextend if necessary to ease insertion.

E. Hyperventilate to assure increased oxygenation.

F. Lift tongue and lower jaw with one hand. Insert the device gently, in the midline down the pharynx with the other hand.

G. Do not force the tube against resistance. If there is difficulty in advancing – redirect, remove and lubricate or remove, reposition head and start again.

H. Seat the device at the proper level with the teeth.

I. Using Combitube (Figure 7-10 and 7-11):

1. Inflate oropharyngeal balloon (#1 blue) with 100 ml of air.

2. Remove syringe and check blue pilot balloon distension.

3. Inflate distal balloon (#2 white) with 10–15 ml air.

4. Remove syringe and check white pilot balloon distension.

5. Ventilate via the longer (#1 blue) connector.

6. Watch for chest rise and auscultate over the stomach to confirm *absence* of air sounds.

   a. If no air sounds over stomach, auscultate breath sounds bilaterally to confirm esophageal placement.

   b. If air sounds are present in stomach, *immediately* disconnect bag from blue (#1) tube and ventilate white (#2) tube.

7. Confirm location and appropriate ventilation. Monitor end-tidal CO_2 if possible.

8. If Combitube is in the esophagus, use port #2 (short white port) for NG suctioning, while ventilating through port #1 (longer blue port).

J. Using PTL airway (Figures 7-12 and 7-13):

1. Adjust neck strap to maintain proper tube depth.

2. Inflate both cuffs by blowing into inflation valve. Assure white cap is on exit valve. May inflate with bag if inflation valve has become contaminated

3. Check pilot balloon distention.

4. Ventilate through #2 short green tube. Watch for chest rise and listen for air sounds over stomach.

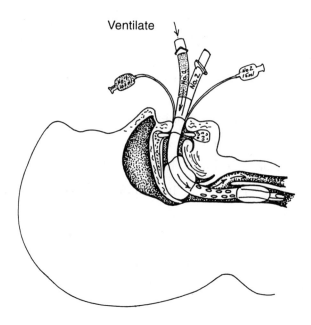

Figure 7-10. Combitube-esophagus

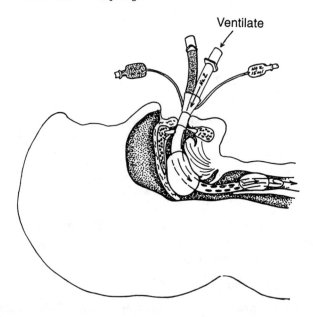

Figure 7-11. Combitube-trachea

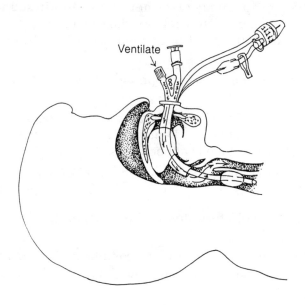

Figure 7-12. PTL esophagus

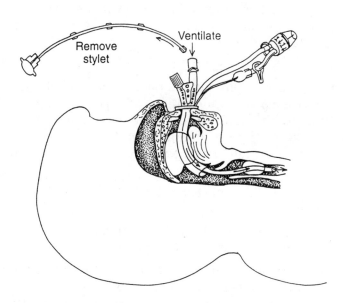

Figure 7-13. PTL trachea

5. Confirm esophageal placement with no air sounds over stomach or immediately remove the stylet from long clear #3 tube and ventilate through #3. Listen to lung sounds bilaterally.

6. Confirm location and appropriate ventilation. Monitor end-tidal CO_2 if possible.

7. Pass NG tube through whichever tube is not being ventilated to decompress stomach. Remove stylet only to pass NG tube if #3 long clear tube is not being used for ventilation.

K. Continue ventilations and monitor end-tidal CO_2, if possible.

Complications

A. Hypoxia, or respiratory death if proper ventilation port not identified.

B. May make transfer of care more complicated if dealing with various levels of training who may not be equally knowledgeable regarding use of the devices.

C. Vomiting and aspiration if removing tube before airway secured with endotracheal tube.

D. Cuffs may tear when inserted in airway with broken teeth, severe mouth trauma or metal dental appliances. Air leaks should be noted and tube replaced.

Special Notes

A. Dual lumen airways are not tolerated in patient with intact gag reflex. Device may need to be removed if patient begins to wake. Unfortunately the gag reflex may return before the patient is really awake enough to handle secretions or even maintain regular respiratory rate. Be particularly cautious in such patients.

B. Endotracheal intubation is possible with the tube in place, but oropharyngeal balloon must be deflated. Stomach contents should be aspirated first.

C. Intubation should always be accomplished before removal of the dual lumen airway in unconscious patients.

D. The advantage of dual lumen airways is also their danger. The provider *must* assess the location of the tube and adjust ventilations appropriately. This encourages thoughtful post-procedure evaluation.

ADVANCED AIRWAY MANAGEMENT: CRICOTHYROTOMY

Introduction

Cricothyrotomy is a difficult and hazardous technique that is to be used only in extraordinary circumstances. This procedure should not be considered a mandatory skill for ALS providers. It is difficult to teach the procedure, and if the paramedic does not practice the procedure often, the skill will not be present to perform the procedure in a timely fashion. Cricothyrotomy produces far more complications than are commonly anticipated.

Indications

Presence of personnel *trained* in the procedure plus inability to establish airway by any other means.

1. Acute upper airway obstruction which cannot be relieved by obstructed airway maneuvers.

2. Upper airway trauma with inability to nasally or orally intubate a patient who has severe respiratory insufficiency.

Precautions

Wear gloves and eye protection.

A. Bleeding is always common, even with correct technique. It should stop once the airway is successfully intubated. Straying from the midline is very dangerous and likely to cause major hemorrhage by injury to the carotid or jugular vessels.

B. Remember that the distance to the carina is very short. Care must be taken not to allow the tube to slip into the right mainstem bronchus if using an endotracheal tube for passage through the cricothyroid space.

C. Standard cricothyrotomy is contra-indicated in children eight years of age and younger because of small cricothyroid space. A needle inserted into that space can still be life saving.

Technique

A. Needle cricothyrotomy:

    1. Equipment

        a. 10, 12 or 14 gauge angiocath.

        b. Oxygen tank with tubing and adapter.

2. Expose the neck.

3. Identify the trachea, palpate the prominent thyroid notch anteriorly. Palpate the cricoid cartilage inferiorly. The space between the cricoid and thyroid cartilages is the cricothyroid space, in which is located the cricothyroid membrane.

4. Stabilize the trachea by holding the thyroid cartilage between thumb and fingers of left hand (if right-handed).

5. Insert the largest available angiocath (14 g or larger) through the skin, just above the cricoid cartilage and pierce the cricothyroid membrane.

6. As soon as the trachea is entered, angle inferiorly and slide needle out as you advance angiocath.

7. Ventilate patient if necessary.

8. Dress wound.

B. Standard cricothyrotomy

1. Equipment:

a. Scalpel and No. 11 blade.

b. Large curved hemostat or extra scalpel handle.

c. Small endotracheal tubes (up to 6 mm in adults) if available.

d. Tracheostomy hook.

e. Tracheal spreader or hemostat.

2. Expose the neck.

3. Identify the trachea, palpate the prominent thyroid notch anteriorly. Palpate the cricoid cartilage inferiorly. The space between the cricoid and thyroid cartilages is the cricothyroid space, in which is located the cricothyroid membrane.

4. Stabilize the trachea by holding the thyroid cartilage between thumb and fingers of left hand (if right-handed).

5. Make a generous vertical incision over the tracheal and cricoid cartilages. Carry the incision down through the platysma and cervical fascia.

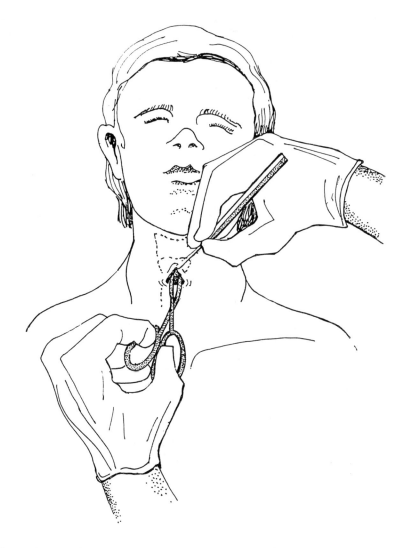

Figure 7-14. Cricothyrotomy with hook and spreader

6. Insert the tracheal hook into the cricoid space and pull the larynx anteriorly into the wound to immobilize it (Figure 7-14).

7. Make a horizontal incision the width of the cricoid anterior space (Figure 7-15).

211

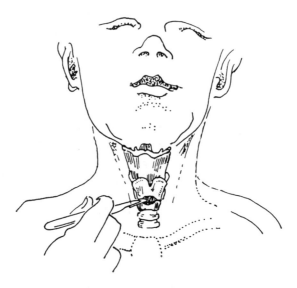

Figure 7-15. Cricothyroid membrane

8. Maintain vertical traction with the tracheostomy hook and dilate the incision. Insert the tracheal spreader or hemostat with the handle directed towards the patient's feet, the tracheal hook being retracted towards the patient's chin.

9. Pass endotracheal tube about 1–1.5 inches into trachea (Figure 7-16).

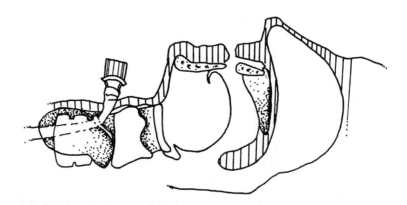

Figure 7-16. Cricothyrotomy – side view

10. Remove the spreader or hemostat and the tracheal hook, being careful not to injure the balloon on the tube.

11. Inflate cuff (if cuffed tube) and ventilate patient with bag, using high flow O_2.

12. Check for breath sounds bilaterally, measure expired CO_2 and secure tube if position is good. It may be impossible to replace if it is coughed or pulled out. It will also easily slide deeper in to the right mainstem bronchus.

13. Control bleeding and dress wound.

14. Suction trachea frequently using sterile technique. Even with inflated balloon, some blood will get into trachea, causing irritation and hypoxia.

Complications
A. Respiratory arrest and patient demise due to:

1. Severity of patient's airway injury.

2. Lack of attention to other potential airway maneuvers.

3. Cricothyrotomy performance which takes too long.

B. Bleeding into airway after cuff insertion with inadequate suctioning.

C. Bleeding within fascial planes of the neck opened during cricothyrotomy.

D. Subcutaneous air due to improper tube or catheter positioning, along with positive ventilation.

E. Bleeding from superficial neck vessels is very common. Use direct pressure after tube is in place.

F. Perforations of the esophagus from penetration by the scalpel.

Special Notes
A. In infants, young children, and many females, the landmarks are less prominent and the thyroid gland is relatively larger, thus making needle cricothyrotomy the preferred procedure.

B. Ventilation through angiocaths is insufficient to provide adequate gas exchange, except briefly, in adults. A needle cricothyrotomy only "buys time" until a definitive procedure can be performed.

C. Although cricothyroid stick and cricothyrotomy are hazardous procedures and have been listed as *direct physician order* procedures, it is apparent that in circumstances where these techniques are actually essential for the patient's airway – there may be no time to make a phone/radio call. In those "time critical" instances, it is better to perform the needed procedure, then document the circumstances in an incident report.

ADVANCED AIRWAY MONITORING: PULSE OXIMETRY

Indications
A. Measurement of the percent of oxygen saturation in the peripheral capillaries.

B. To assist with determining the optimal amount of supplemental oxygen to administer. May be particularly useful in patients with COPD or other chronic respiratory diseases.

C. To help differentiate various causes of shortness of breath.

Precautions
A. Do not rely on any single device to make patient care decisions.

B. Oxygen saturation does not reflect work of breathing. Patients with adequate oxygen saturation can work so hard to achieve that saturation that they may experience abrupt respiratory failure or arrest from fatigue.

C. Some patients with chronic lung disease do not normally have an oxygen saturation greater than 90%. If titrating oxygen doses to keep the saturation above 90%, this small group of patients may slow their drive to breathe and may actually stop breathing. Be ready to support ventilation if this occurs.

D. Patients with poor peripheral perfusion (hypovolemic shock, severe vasoconstriction from hypothermia or other conditions) may not have enough digital circulation to give accurate pulse oximetry readings. Be sure the wave form varies with pulses. Monitoring the ear lobe may be preferable in those patients.

E. Saturation percentages do not reflect the actual content of oxygen in a linear fashion. Once the saturation is less than 80%, oxygen content can drop precipitously with very small changes in lung function.

F. In carbon monoxide poisoning, saturation measurements are normal because the disabled hemoglobin is counted as normal oxygenated hemoglobin by the sensor. Likewise, in a severely anemic patient, the *amount* of hemoglobin available to carry oxygen is the problem, while the saturation of the hemoglobin that is active is normal.

Technique

A. Turn on oximetry machine.

B. Attach sensor probe to fingertip, toe or earlobe.

C. Secure with tape if needed.

D. Observe for a pulsing wave form to assure adequate perfusion. Confirm that pulse rate equals your measurement of this vital sign.

E. Adjust probe to get a clear waveform.

F. Document saturation when level stabilizes.

Complications

A. This is a non-invasive device without complications except time wasted or distraction from observation of the patient whose work of breathing is the critical problem.

B. May produce false reassurance in patients with some hemoglobinopathies (carboxyhemoglobin or fetal hemoglobin) who may be quite hypoxic and have normal pulse oximetry readings.

Special Notes

A. Normal oxygen saturation is between 95–99%. Patients with saturations less than 90% should receive oxygen until their saturation is at the 90% level, if possible. COPD patients may be comfortable at lower levels.

B. Fingernail polish may need to be removed to give an accurate pulse oximetry reading, since the reading is based on sensing color differences between oxyhemoglobin (red) and reduced hemoglobin (blue).

ADVANCED AIRWAY MONITORING: CAPNOGRAPHY

Indications
A. To confirm tube placement immediately after endotracheal intubation in a patient with pulse or respiratory effort.

B. As an additional evaluation tool for the patient in cardiac arrest who is intubated with either an endotracheal tube or a dual lumen airway.

C. To monitor endotracheal tube placement during transport to assure that tube location does not change.

Precautions
A. End-tidal CO_2 monitoring is an excellent adjunctive tool to assess the location of the endotracheal tube and the response of the cardiovascular and pulmonary system. It is not a substitute for the most important technique to assure accurate intubation, which is direct visualization of the vocal cords during placement of the endotracheal tube.

B. End-tidal CO_2 values must be interpreted with caution in the patient who is in full cardiac arrest. In the absence of effective circulation the value will be low or zero even with successful tracheal intubation. If the tube was seen to pass through the cords . and equal breaths sounds are heard, capnography can be delayed or even eliminated in the cardiac arrest patient.

Technique
A. After intubation attach probe in-line at the end of the endotracheal tube.

B. Note lighting or flash of any color change to confirm correct positioning in the airway.

C. Document confirmation evidence in the patient report (verbal and written).

Complications
A. This is a noninvasive procedure without complications other than time delays created by obtaining readings when more critical care of the patient is warranted.

B. Time delays may also result from misinterpretation of low expired CO_2 from low flow state rather than incorrect placement of the tube.

Special Notes

A. End-tidal CO_2 colorimetric measures can be made useless by moisture. Under ideal circumstances they produce measurements comparable to the capnometers. That may not always be true in field use.

B. There is some data available that false positive results can be created by carbonated beverages bubbling CO_2 from the stomach. It seems unlikely that this should cause a significant clinical error, but it is important to remember – capnography is just another "gadget" which should not replace clinical assessment.

C. As noted previously, the end-tidal CO_2 measurement in the cardiac arrest patient can be difficult to interpret. After correct intubation, however, there is some data to suggest that patients with sufficient circulation to produce levels of CO_2 of 15 torr, or greater, are more likely to have a return of pulse and respirations than patients with levels of 5 torr or less. Presumably the longer the down time and the lower the end-tidal CO_2, the less likely the resuscitation will be successful. Certainly no one is advocating the use for predicting success (or failure) in the field, but it may be an additional clue in those patients who do not seem to be responding to all of the usual medications.

BANDAGING

Indications

A. To stop external bleeding by application of direct and continuous pressure to wound site.

B. To protect patient from contamination to lacerations, abrasions, burns.

C. To prevent heat loss from burn area in major burn victims.

Precautions

Wear gloves and eye protection.

A. Although external skin wounds may be dramatic, they are rarely a high management priority in the trauma victim.

B. Do not use circumferential dressings around neck. Continued swelling may block airway.

C. Wounds containing large amounts of clotted blood may not stop bleeding readily. Gently remove the clots with sterile gauze or irrigating saline before dressing the wound.

Equipment

1000 ml normal saline for irrigation
Dressings:
    4×4 inch sterile gauze material
    large absorbent sterile dressing material (Universal dressing)
Bandages:
    self-adherent gauze materials (rolled)
    clean cloths or triangular bandages, tape

Technique

A. Stop exsanguinating hemorrhage with direct pressure. Use clean cloth or dressing.

B. Assess patient fully and treat all injuries by priority once assessment is complete.

C. Remove gross dirt and contamination from wound – remove clothing if easily removable, rinse dirt, gasoline, acids, or alkalis. Use copious irrigating saline or tap water for chemical contamination.

D. Evaluate wound for depth, presence of fracture in wound, foreign body, or evidence of injury to deep structures. Note distal motor, sensory, and circulatory function prior to applying dressings.

E. Apply sterile dressing to wound surface. Touch outer side of dressing only.

F. Apply splint or PASG over dressing if needed.

G. Wrap dressing with clean gauze or cloth bandages, applied just tightly enough to hold dressing securely (if no splint applied).

H. Assess wound for evidence of continued bleeding.

I. Check distal pulses, color, capillary refill, and sensation after bandage applied.

J. Continue to apply direct hand pressure over dressing or use air splint if bleeding not controlled with bandage alone.

Complications
A. Loss of distal circulation from bandage applied too tightly around extremity. Do not use elastic bandages nor apply bandages too tightly for this reason.

B. Airway obstruction due to tight circumferential neck bandage.

C. Restriction of breathing from circumferential chest wound splinting.

D. Continued bleeding no longer visible under dressings. (This is particularly common with scalp wounds which continue to lose large amounts of unnoticed blood. Remember to clean out clots and matted hair, if possible before dressing wound.)

E. Inadequate hemostasis – some wounds require continuous direct manual pressure to stop bleeding.

Special Notes
A. An excellent paramedic once said that he bandaged patients as the ambulance was backing into the hospital entrance – he knew that the bandaging was often the least important of his functions but wanted the patient to look neat for all of us. There is a lot to be said for this approach – and even for leaving the bandages off entirely in critical patients.

B. When several levels of responders treat the patient at the scene, bandages by the first responders may impair the ability of other prehospital personnel to assess the patient fully. This dilemma must be worked through for every system. Either significant wounds should be covered temporarily by first responders or a good relationship between crews should be established so that the answerable person knows whether the wound dressed by a first responder is an open fracture, a deep wound with probable injury to deep structures, or just a superficial wound.

C. In situations where premade bandaging materials are not available, improvise! Only dressings, those materials which are applied directly to the wound, need to be sterile. If sterile materials are not available, the cleanest cloth with the least amount of lint and contamination should be used.

CARDIOVERSION

By direct physician order only.

Indications
A. Use only *in emergency situations* where there is a rapid rhythm associated with inadequate cardiac output and signs of poor perfusion (confusion, coma, angina, systolic BP < 90 mm Hg):

1. Ventricular tachycardia

2. Supraventricular tachycardia (PSVT, acute atrial fibrillation, or atrial flutter)

3. Unknown – wide complex (ventricular vs. supraventricular) tachycardia.

B. Contra-indicated when digitalis toxicity is cause of rhythm. When patient is decompensating and you suspect digitalis toxicity, give bolus of lidocaine before cardioverting and start at lowest machine setting (5 joules if possible).

Precautions
A. Precautions for defibrillation apply. Protect rescuers!

B. A patient who is talking to you is probably perfusing adequately. He will remember a cardioversion for a long time – and so will you!

C. If the defibrillator does not discharge on "synch" with tachycardia, turn off "synch" button and refire. The waves may not have enough amplitude to trigger the synch mechanism.

D. If sinus rhythm is achieved, even transiently, with cardioversion, subsequent cardioversion at a *higher* energy setting will be of no additional value. Leave the setting the same, consider correction of hypoxia, acidosis, etc., to hold the conversion.

E. If the patient is pulseless, begin CPR and treat as cardiac arrest, even if the electrical rhythm appears organized (see PEA).

Technique
A. Administer O_2, high flow (10–15 L/min) by mask.

B. Start IV prior to procedure – D5W, TKO.

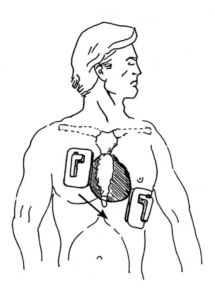

Figure 7-17. Paddle placement

C. Assemble resuscitation equipment – suction, bag-valve-mask, NP or OP airways, laryngoscope, intubation tubes.

D. Premedicate with diazepam if patient alert.

E. Attach monitor and select lead that gives upright QRS complex.

F. Turn synchronizer switch to "on" position.

G. Set charge at 100 joules.

H. Charge defibrillator.

I. Place electrode jelly on paddles.

J. Apply paddles to chest as for defibrillation (Figure 7-17).

K. Hold firing buttons depressed until synchronizer fires defibrillator.

L. If no firing occurs and patient is in wide complex tachycardia, turn off "synch" switch and refire.

M. If firing occurs but rhythm does not convert, turn machine up in 100 joule increments and refire as needed.

N. If patient is cardioverted into or progresses to ventricular fibrillation, immediately:

1. Increase charge to defibrillation level (200–300 joules).

2. Recharge defibrillator.

3. Turn off "synch" switch.

4. Defibrillate.

Complications

A. Erythema or irritation of skin will occur, particularly if good lubrication and skin contact are not achieved.

B. Muscle cramps and pain in awake patient.

C. Ventricular fibrillation and asystole occur rarely and usually in the digitalis-toxic patient.

Special Notes

A. Cardioversion is *rarely* indicated in children.

B. Tachycardias are particularly devastating in patient with artificial valves which cannot move fast.

C. People with chronic atrial fibrillation are very difficult to convert and their atrial fibrillation is not usually the cause of their decompensation. If you get a history of "irregular heartbeat", look elsewhere for the problem.

D. Sinus tachycardia can occur up to 160–180 beats/minute. It is a *symptom* of an underlying problem. The patient must be treated for the underlying cause. Cardioversion is *not* indicated. Initial treatment should be as for shock if perfusion is poor.

E. IV diazepam (5–10 mg in adult) may be used in conscious patients prior to cardioversion, but field cardioversion is not usually indicated in this case. Discuss with base if you feel diazepam is indicated.

F. Do not be overly concerned about the dysrhythmias that normally occur in the few minutes following successful cardioversion. These usually respond to time and adequate oxygenation and should only be treated if they persist more than 5 minutes.

CAROTID SINUS MASSAGE

By direct physician order only.

Indications
A. Treatment of supraventricular tachycardia with signs of hypoperfusion (decreased level of consciousness, angina, BP < 90 mm Hg, congestive heart failure *caused* by tachycardia).

B. Treatment of tachycardia of unknown etiology (supraventricular vs. ventricular) with signs of hypoperfusion.

C. To determine etiology of supraventricular tachycardias (for field use ONLY with signs of hypoperfusion).

Tachycardia	Expected Response to CSM
Sinus tachycardia	no response or gradual slowing
Paroxysmal supraventricular tachycardia (PSVT)	no response or sudden conversion to NSR
Atrial flutter	increased block, ventricular slowing, revealing flutter waves
Atrial fibrillation	variable slowing
Ventricular tachycardia	no response

Precautions
A. Never occlude both carotid arteries at once. Your patient may lose all circulation to the brain.

B. CSM stimulates the baroreceptor in the carotid sinus which, in turn, produces vagal stimulation to the heart. Since the vagus innervates only the atria and the A-V node, no effect will be seen in ventricular dysrhythmias.

Technique
A. Apply monitor electrodes.

B. IV, saline lock or D5W, TKO.

C. Document rhythm with paper recording (or telemetry).

D. Explain procedure to patient.

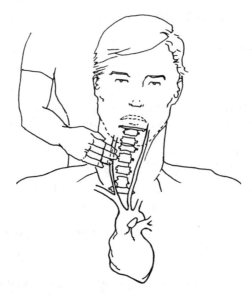

Figure 7-18. Carotid sinus massage

E. Attempt Valsalva maneuver first, if possible. Patient should "bear down" against closed glottis, 20–30 seconds.

F. Lie patient down (if tolerated), expose neck by removing clothing and hyperextending slightly.

G. Gently palpate for carotid pulses on one side, then the other. Proceed only if bilateral carotid pulses are felt.

H. Apply pressure to right carotid artery, gently massaging the superior end, just below the mandible (Figure 7-18) (locate pulse just medial to the angle of the mandible). Pressure should not obstruct carotid flow but should be firm.

I. Monitor rhythm constantly throughout procedure.

J. Release massage immediately if:

    1. Patient becomes confused and shows signs of brain ischemia.

    2. Any slowing or pause in heart rate occurs.

    3. 15 seconds of massage has been completed.

K. If CSM slows rhythm, document by paper recording.

L. If asystole occurs and persists for longer than 15 seconds:

1. Initiate CPR, administer chest thump.

2. Administer atropine 1.0 mg IV.

3. Proceed as per Asystole Protocol.

M. If no response to CSM, allow patient to rest for 2–4 minutes, then re-attempt massage using left carotid artery.

N. Notify base physician for further orders. If indicated, lidocaine or cardioversion may be considered.

O. Continue to monitor cardiac rhythm closely during 5 minutes following release of carotid sinus pressure.

Complications

A. Asystole.

B. Stroke from dislodged carotid artery thrombus in persons with atherosclerotic disease.

C. Brain ischemia from improper CSM causing occlusion of carotid artery or compromise of marginally perfused areas of brain.

Special Notes

A. It is difficult to differentiate congestive heart failure (CHF) caused by tachycardia from a tachycardia caused by CHF. Pulse rates under 160 are usually secondary rather than the primary problem.

B. CSM is not a field procedure to be used on awake, alert patients. In these patients, documentation, diagnosis, and treatment should be left to the receiving physician. Field CSM is indicated only when hypoperfusion, angina, or circulatory compromise result from the dysrhythmia and transport time justifies added time delay.

C. Dysrhythmias are likewise common after conversion of rhythms by CSM. Treatment is indicated only if persistent > 5 minutes.

D. Always check for presence of good pulses in *both* carotids (particularly in elderly patients) prior to attempting massage on one carotid.

DEFIBRILLATION

Indications
A. Ventricular fibrillation by monitor.

B. Ventricular tachycardia in the pulseless and unconscious patient.

Precautions
A. Do not treat the monitor strip alone. Treat the patient! A patient who is talking is *not* in ventricular fibrillation, whatever the monitor shows. Artifact can commonly simulate ventricular fibrillation.

B. Dry the chest wall if wet. Do not drip saline or electrode jelly across the chest. This results in bridging, which conducts the current through the skin rather than through the heart.

C. Nitroglycerin paste, which is commonly used by cardiac patients, is flammable and may ignite if not wiped from the chest prior to paddle contact.

D. Defibrillation should be accompanied by visible muscle contraction by patient. If this does not occur, the paddles did not discharge. Recheck equipment.

E. Unsuccessful defibrillation is often due to hypoxia or acidosis. Careful attention to airway management and proper CPR is important.

F. Protect rescuers – *"clear"* the area!

Technique
A. Establish unresponsiveness.

B. Open airway, check for breathing and initiate CPR.

C. Maintain CPR with 1 or 2 rescuers.

D. Second or third person should get monitor-defibrillator and turn it on.

E. Place conductive gel on paddles.

F. Place "quick look" paddles in appropriate position to determine rhythm. Obtain print-out if possible.

G. Stop CPR and evaluate rhythm (5–10 seconds maximum). If ventricular fibrillation is present, continue with protocol. Otherwise, see Cardiac Arrest Protocol.

H. Resume CPR.

I. Check synchronizer switch "off".

J. Charge defibrillator with paddles in hand:

Adult – 200 joules delivered energy.

Child – 2 joules/Kg or 1 joule/pound.

K. Place paddles with as much anterior/posterior direction of current as possible. One paddle just to the right of the upper sternum and below the clavicle and the other just to the left of the apex, or just to the left of the left nipple in the anterior axillary line. Use twist to distribute conductive gel evenly on chest wall.

L. Recheck rhythm. "Clear" the area.

M. Apply firm pressure (about 25 lb) to paddles. Be careful not to lean and let paddles slip off.

N. Press defibrillator buttons. Watch for muscle contraction. Leave paddles in place to check rhythm.

O. If ventricular fibrillation persists, immediately recharge and reshock at 200–300 joules.

P. If organized rhythm appears, check pulse.

Q. If no pulse, resume CPR and continue with Cardiac Arrest protocol.

Complications
A. Rescuer defibrillation may occur if you forget to clear the area or lean against metal stretcher or patient during the procedure.

B. Skin burns result from inadequate electrode gel on paddles and chest, or from inadequate contact between paddles and skin.

C. Damage to the heart muscle is directly related to amount of energy which is run through it. The lower defibrillation charges are recommended to minimize myocardial damage but still provide maximum chance of defibrillating the heart.

Special Notes
A. Defibrillation is not the first step in treating fibrillation due to traumatic hypovolemia. CPR and fluid resuscitation is first.

B. Defibrillation may not be successful in ventricular fibrillation due to hypothermia until the core temperature is above 88 degrees Fahrenheit (31 degrees Centigrade). Attempt to defibrillate, but prolonged CPR during rewarming may be necessary before conversion is possible.

C. Knowledge of your defibrillator is important! Delivered energy varies with different machines. Make sure your machine is maintained regularly. Testing with full discharge is recommended weekly. Low energy discharge is recommended daily (a periodic full discharge can also improve battery performance). A chart should be attached to the machine listing actual delivered energy for usual energy levels.

D. Dysrhythmias are common following successful defibrillation. They respond to time and oxygenation. Treat only if persisting > 5 minutes.

FOLEY CATHETER INSERTION

By direct physician order during long transports only.

Indications
In unconscious patients being treated with mannitol or furosemide when transport time is sufficiently long that patient is at risk for bladder rupture. Also prevents spills and contamination from incontinence.

Precautions
Wear gloves and eye protection.

A. Contraindicated in patients with bleeding from the urinary meatus.

B. Relatively contraindicated in the presence of pelvic or abdominal trauma. An attempt may be made to pass the catheter but extreme caution must be exercised. Keep a high index of suspicion that trauma to the urinary tract may exist. If any resistance is felt during insertion, procedure must be discontinued.

C. Do not inflate balloon without free flow of urine.

Technique
A. Assemble equipment and explain procedure to patient if conscious. (Prepackaged Foley catheter insertion set is preferred.)

B. Drape and position patient, preferably in frog-leg position, exposing perineum.

C. Wash hands.

D. Open tray.

E. Put on sterile gloves.

F. Poor antiseptic over cotton balls.

G. Place underpad under buttocks with absorbent side up.

H. Lift plastic tray from carton and place on underpad.

I. Unfold fenestrated drape and cover area around genitalia.

J. Open lubricant and squeeze onto underpad.

K. In female:

    1. Separate labia gently with thumb and forefinger, spread out and up *(this glove is contaminated and will remain in this position during procedure)*.

    2. Using forceps to hold absorbent cotton balls, use one at a time with single downward stroke and cleanse the far side of

exposed area, near and then directly over meatus. Repeat several times. Discard cotton balls.

3. Position catheter tray between patient's thighs.

4. With uncontaminated hand, pick up the catheter at least 3 inches from tip (Figure 7-19). Lubricate.

5. Identify meatus. Insert catheter gently (Figure 7-20). *Never force.*

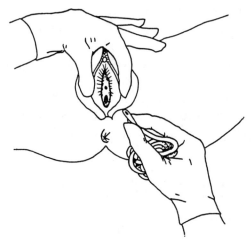

Figure 7-19. Female catheterization

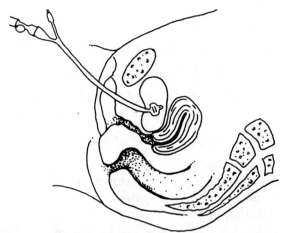

Figure 7-20. Female catheter in place

L. In male:

1. With one hand, grasp the penis and hold it securely. If there is foreskin, it should be gently retracted as you grasp penis and held back to prevent it from contaminating area around meatus (Figure 7-21) *(this glove is now contaminated and will remain in this position during procedure)*.

2. Wash glans (or meatus) of penis with saturated absorbent cotton balls. Begin with meatus and wipe glans with circular motion. Repeat several times. Discard cotton balls.

3. Hold penis forward and slightly upward to stretch urethra.

4. With uncontaminated hand, pick up the catheter at least 3 inches from tip. Lubricate.

5. Insert about 7 inches (Figure 7-22), touching the tubing to be inserted as little as possible while inserting.

6. To assist insertion, ask patient to try to void if conscious. Changing the angle of traction on the penis may also assist in insertion.

M. Insert catheter 3–4 inches after first urine flow.

N. Inflate balloon with prefilled syringe (if discomfort or resistance, deflate, advance further and reinflate).

O. Withdraw catheter slightly (and gently) to be sure balloon is inflated.

P. Attach catheter to drainage set.

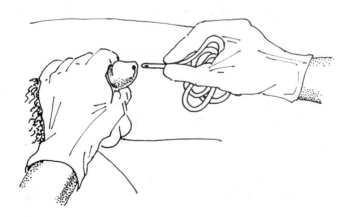

Figure 7-21. Male catheterization

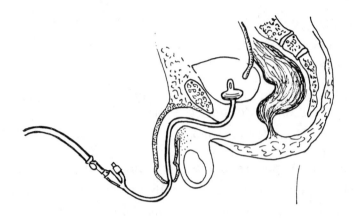

Figure 7-22. Male catheter in place

Q. Tape catheter firmly to anterior thigh. This tape should absorb all traction forces on the system. No traction should exist on the catheter or balloon itself.

R. Recheck drainage system for leaks.

S. Dry area.

T. Remove drapes and make patient comfortable.

U. Do not raise bag above bladder level if possible.

Complications
A. Forcing the catheter in the presence of a urethral tear can create a false channel and increase the injury.

B. Infection due to poor technique is common.

Special Notes
A. Return of grossly bloody fluid without resistance does not mean you must stop the procedure, as long as it has been otherwise normal and you feel reasonably sure you are in the bladder. Notify base physician.

B. If, for any reason, the catheter is to be removed, remember to deflate the balloon *prior* to gently withdrawing the catheter.

IMPLANTABLE CARDIOVERTER DEFIBRILLATOR (ICD) MAGNET

Indications
ICD device that is generating inappropriate shocks (usually shocking sinus tachycardia or PSVT rather than ventricular tachycardia or ventricular fibrillation).

Precautions
A. Patient may be understandably quite anxious and difficult to evaluate. The call will usually be for a defibrillator that "keeps going off". The majority of the time this will be because the patient is having frequent episodes of unstable ventricular tachycardia. Occasionally however, the device will be abnormally sensing a sinus or supraventricular tachycardia. Careful monitoring will allow the paramedic to differentiate these scenarios.

   It is inappropriate to "turn off" an ICD that is properly sensing and treating dysrhythmias.

B. In a patient who is determined to have an ICD device which is sensing and inappropriately shocking, full resuscitation equipment must be available before using the magnet to "turn off" the ICD.

Technique
A. Obtain full history including brand or name of ICD device that has been implanted (Figure 7-23).

B. Apply O_2, moderate flow (4–6 L/min).

C. IV, D5W, TKO.

D. Attach cardiac monitor.

E. Record rhythm and any defibrillations if possible.

F. If rhythm inappropriate for internal defibrillation, assure external defibrillator and intubation equipment are readily available. Use ICD magnet to turn device off. Magnet response is device specific:

   1. CPI (1500, 1550, 1600) – placing the magnet over the device will cause the device to beep with each R wave it senses (Figure 7-24). If left in place for 30 seconds an audible continuous tone means the device is *off*. Remove magnet to keep the device off.

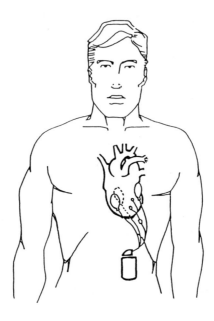

Figure 7-23. ICD in abdominal wall

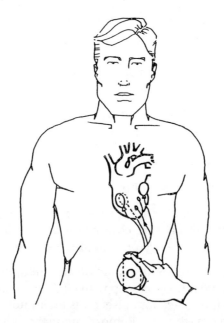

Figure 7-24. Magnet over end of ICD

2. CPI (PRX) – has a programmable magnet function that will allow a magnet to suspend detection if programmed *on* and have no effect if programmed *off*.

3. Ventritex (Cadence) – magnet will suspend detection and therapy (no therapies/shocks will be delivered) while magnet is over either end of the device. Detections will resume when magnet is removed. There is no audible tone with magnet placement. V-100 series may be programmed to ignore the application of a magnet.

4. Intermedics (ResQ) – magnet will suspend detections while in place. Detection will resume (with programmed therapies) if magnet is removed.

5. Ventak PRx (1700/1705) – has a programmable magnet function that will allow a magnet to suspend detection if programmed *on* and have no effect if programmed *off*. If magnet use is programmed *on* place the magnet over the pulse generator and listen for tones from the device. The pulse generator is *off* or *monitor only* if a continuous tone is heard. The pulse generator is in monitor + therapy if it emits tones synchronously with each R-wave (it will suspend therapy while magnet in place and resume when magnet removed). An absence of tones indicates the device is not sensing.

6. Medtronic PCD (7219/7202) – has a programmable magnet function, as above. If programmed *on* the device will temporarily suspend detection and therapy functions when the magnet is in place over the ICD device.

G. Continue to monitor closely and transport to appropriate facility (preferably where the patient had the ICD device implanted).

H. Be prepared to defibrillate if ICD has been turned off. If necessary to defibrillate, *anterior-posterior patch placement is preferred*. Sternum-apex paddle or patch placement may damage lead wires from ICD.

Complications

A. Since some devices react differently to the magnet, it is important to be sure which ICD device has been implanted. The device may still be functional though you think you have turned it off. Most of these patients will have histories of documented ventricular fibrillation or tachycardia associated with sudden death or symptomatic sustained ventricular tachycardia. The patient and their family will usually be quite well educated on the ICD device. They should have written material and may even have a magnet in the home.

B. Once you have used the magnet to turn the device off, the patient is at your mercy for further care. Assure all ACLS equipment is available before turning the ICD device off.

Special Notes

A. Patients will frequently be quite frantic if the ICD device has fired several times. They will be most anxious for the paramedic to turn off the device. Use caution! If the device is firing appropriately you will be replacing a 5–10 joule internal shock for a 200–360 joule external shock. The patient will not be pleased with the change.

B. The magnet will also effect pacemakers, but is not recommended for field use on pacemakers.

C. Contact with patient will not be deleterious to field personnel. CPR should continue normally if so indicated. ACLS protocols should also be followed as usual. Shocks can be delivered from ICD and external devices if so indicated without effect on the ICD device. *Watch for rhythm.*

INTRAOSSEOUS CANNULATION

Indications
Critical child, less than six years of age, in need of emergent fluids or medications and in whom at least one IV has been attempted without success.

Precautions
Wear gloves and eye protection.

A. One puncture of the bone will allow any subsequent punctures to leak fluid from the initial puncture. Thus, no more than one attempt at one site should be used in the field.

B. Many medications have been reported given by the intraosseous route, however, the data are still not available to determine the efficacy or safety with certainty. Medications that have been approved for endotracheal instillation should probably be given via ET tube when possible.

Technique
A. Equipment:

   1. 18 gauge spinal needle, 15g bone marrow needle, or standard intraosseous needle.

   2. 10–20 ml syringe filled with RL or NS.

   3. IV connecting tubing.

B. Support lower extremity with knee flexed slightly over towel.

C. *Scrub* insertion site. (Betadine vs. alcohol is less important than vigor).

D. Insert needle through skin to anterior surface of tibia, 2–3 cm distal to tibial tuberosity.

E. Insert needle into bone marrow cavity with twisting motion (Figure 7-25). Needle should be directed perpendicularly or slightly inferiorly to avoid the epiphyseal plate (Figure 7-26).

F. Needle will be felt to "pop" into marrow cavity. It should then stand upright without assistance and fluid should flow easily.

G. Support needle with dressing and tape.

H. Attach IV connecting tube filled with fluid and inject 20 ml/kg, if needed. (Medications may also be administered, under direct physician order.)

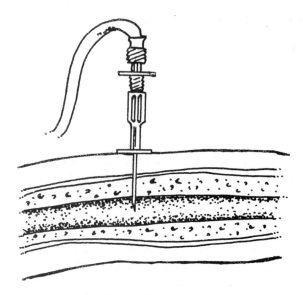

Figure 7-25. Intraosseous needle – side view

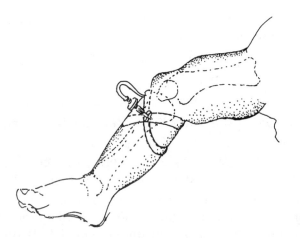

Figure 7-26. Intraosseous needle and line in position

Complications
A. As noted, fluid will extrude from any previous bony intrusions, or from through-and-through penetration of the bone. This will result in injection of fluid into tissues of the leg which should not be dangerous but will not be very effective use of fluids.

B. Infections of bony structures have been reported and are very significant problems in young children. Good cleansing techniques and short term use of this temporary measure will minimize the risk.

Special Notes

A. Some authorities recommend aspiration of marrow fluid or tissue to confirm needle location. This is not recommended for field procedures as it increases the risk of plugging the needle.

B. Although this technique is appropriate for standing order in children who are in cardiorespiratory arrest, it should be utilized in other children only after direct physician communication.

C. All medications administered via intraosseous route need to be given by direct physician order only.

D. This technique is currently recommended by the American Heart Association for Pediatric Advanced Life Support. The course in its entirety is recommended, but the technique for intraosseous infusion may be learned separately.

MEDICATION ADMINISTRATION

Indications
Illness or injury which requires medication to improve or maintain the patient's condition.

Precautions
Wear gloves and eye protection.

A. Certain medications can be administered via one route only, others via several. If you are uncertain about the drug you are giving – check with base station.

B. Make certain that the medication you want to give is the one in your hand. Always double check medication and dose before administration.

C. IM and SQ routes are unpredictable – medications are absorbed erratically via these routes and may not be absorbed at all if the patient is seriously ill and severely vasoconstricted. The IV route should be used almost exclusively in the field. If an IV cannot be started, the endotracheal and rectal routes are the best alternatives.

Technique
A. Use syringe just large enough to hold appropriate quantity of medication (or use prefilled syringe).

B. Attach large gauge needle (19–21 gauge) to syringe.

C. Break ampule or cleanse multi-dose vial with alcohol (the latter is less desirable for field use).

D. Using sterile technique, draw medication into syringe.

E. Change needles to small gauge (21 gauge or smaller) for IM or SQ.

Intravenous injection technique
A. Use needle appropriate for viscosity of fluid injected. Glucose requires larger gauge needle (19 gauge). For most other medications, 20 gauge or smaller is appropriate.

B. Cleanse IV tubing injection site with alcohol.

C. Check medication in hand – confirm medication, dose, and amount.

D. Eject air from syringe.

E. Insert needle into injection site.

F. Pinch IV tubing closed between bottle and needle.

G. Inject at a rate which is appropriate for the medication.

H. Withdraw needle and release tubing to restore flow.

I. Record medication given, dose, amount, and time.

Endotracheal injection technique
A. Prepare medication to be given and set next to patient being ventilated.

B. Ventilate fully and rapidly 4–5 times prior to disconnecting the bag from the endotracheal tube.

C. Check medication in hand. Confirm medication, dose, and amount.

D. Endotracheal dose is generally 2–2$^1/_2$ times the IV dose. (Endotracheal dose of epinephrine for pediatric arrest is 10 times the IV dose.) Dilute in 5–10 ml NS.

E. Administer half the appropriate dose into the endotracheal tube.

F. Connect the bag and ventilate rapidly an additional 4–5 times.

G. Disconnect bag and administer the remaining half of medication into endotracheal tube.

H. Again connect the self-inflating bag and ventilate rapidly 4–5 times before resuming the recommended ventilation rate according to the age and condition of patient.

I. Record medication given, dose, amount and time.

Intramuscular injection technique
For use only by physician order in special situations.

A. Use long 21–22 gauge needle (1–1.5").

B. Check medication in hand – confirm medication, dose and amount.

C. Select injection site (usually deltoid, but may be upper outer quadrant of gluteus if more convenient).

D. Cleanse site.

E. Eject air from syringe.

F. Stretch skin over injection site.

G. Insert needle through skin into muscle, aspirate and, if no blood return, inject medication.

H. Remove needle and put pressure over injection site with sterile swab.

I. Record medication given, dose, amount, and time.

Subcutaneous injection technique
For use only by physician order.

A. Use 25 gauge needle 5/8" length for most subcutaneous injections.

B. Check medication in hand – confirm medication, dose, and amount.

C. Select injection site (usually just distal and posterior to deltoid).

D. Cleanse site.

E. Eject air from syringe.

F. Insert needle perpendicularly to hilt (5/8" only).

G. Aspirate and, if there is no blood return, inject medication.

H. Remove needle and put pressure over injection site with sterile swab.

I. Record medication given, dose, amount, and time.

Nebulization technique

A. Use hand-held nebulizer with mouthpiece (or mask for patient unable to hold mouthpiece).

B. Check medication in hand. Confirm medication, dose, and amount.

C. Draw up dose of medication in syringe or dropper – inject into nebulizer chamber. Add unit dose directly.

D. Add diluent, if needed (usually water or NS) in appropriate amount to chamber.

E. Attach to O_2 tubing and set at 6–8 L/min (sufficient to produce good vaporization).

F. Administer for approximately 5 minutes, until solution gone from chamber.

G. Record medication given, dose, amount, and time.

Intraosseous technique
A. Prepare medication to be administered.

B. Check medication in hand – confirm medication, dose, and amount.

C. Inject into port on intraosseous line, or . . .

D. Remove needle from syringe and inject directly into intraosseous needle.

E. Record medication given, dose, amount, and time.

Rectal technique
For use only by physician order in special situations.

A. Prepare medication to be administered.

B. Check medication in hand – confirm medication, dose, and amount.

C. Aspirate medication into 1–2 ml syringe *with no needle.*

D. Lubricate the tip of the syringe with water soluble lubricant.

E. Insert the tip of the syringe into the rectum, just past the sphincter muscle (approximately one cm).

F. Inject the medication.

G. Remove the syringe and hold legs and buttocks together for 1–2 minutes.

H. Record medication given, dose, amount, and time.

Complications
A. Local extravasation during IV medication injection, particularly with calcium or dextrose, may cause tissue necrosis. Watch carefully and be ready to stop injection immediately.

B. Allergic and anaphylactic reactions occur more rapidly with IV injections, but may occur with medication administered by any route.

C. Too rapid IV injection can cause untoward side effects. For example, diazepam can cause apnea and epinephrine can cause asystole or severe hypertension.

D. IM or SQ injection causes uncertain medication levels over time. Later treatment may be jeopardized because of slow release and later effects of medication given hours before.

Special Notes
A. Several medications are carried in different concentrations in an emergency medical kit. Be sure you are using the correct concentration! Epinephrine 1:10,000 and 1:1,000 are the most common to confuse.

B. Carry pediatric drugs in a separate area of the drug case.

C. Endotracheal medication administration provides onset of drug effect almost as rapidly as with IV administration. The action is more sustained, though, so, for example, epinephrine given via ET tube is not repeated every 5 minutes as an IV dose is.

D. Administration of medication rectally is probably only going to be used for children with status seizures in whom IV access may be very difficult. The effects are almost as rapid as IV and there is an equal chance for respiratory depression – be prepared to assist ventilation before administration of diazepam.

NASOGASTRIC INTUBATION

By direct physician order for long transports only.

Indications
A. Relief of gastric distention.
B. Relief of vomiting from various causes during transport or transfer.
C. Relief of abdominal pain caused by solid organ diseases (e.g., pancreatitis, cholecystitis).
D. To empty and irrigate stomach with upper GI bleeding.

Precautions
Wear gloves and eye protection.

A. Contraindicated with facial fractures or nasal bleeding.
B. Contraindicated with potential for upper airway obstructions (foreign body, epiglottitis).
C. If endotracheal tube is in place, cuff may need to be released before tube will pass through esophagus.

Technique
A. Equipment:

1. Nasogastric tube:

   0–1 year – 6–8 French feeding tube.

   1–5 years – 8–10 Salem sump or Levin tube.

   5–15 years – 10–14 Salem sump or Levin tube.

   >15 years – 16–18 Salem sump or Levin tube.

2. Emesis basin or rubber glove for passive drainage.
3. Irrigation syringe for intermittent suction or periodic saline irrigation.
4. Xylocaine jelly or Lubafax for less painful insertion and prevention of epistaxis.

B. Have patient sitting or semi-upright if possible. Keep head in midline. Explain procedure to patient.
C. Measure tube length before insertion – nose to ear to xiphoid process. (Usually corresponds to second black line on standard adult tube.)

D. Lubricate tube.

E. Gently insert through one nostril (left is most useful if not occluded by septal deformity). Angle tube *horizontally* or slightly downward.

F. Have patient swallow as he feels the tube in the back of the throat. Slight neck flexion with patient sitting forward provides best positioning.

G. Continue passage to correct length (Figure 7-27). If tubing coils in back of throat, remove enough to straighten then reattempt passage.

H. After insertion, listen over epigastrium as air is injected through tube via irrigation syringe (10–20 ml). If bubbling is heard, apply suction to syringe. Gastric content may be clear, blood flecked, yellow-green (bile-stained) or brown (coffee ground appearance from blood in acid medium).

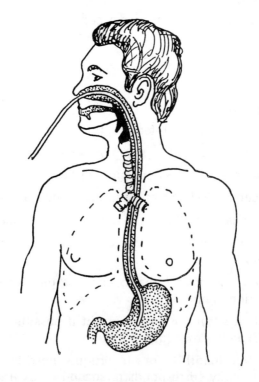

Figure 7-27. Nasogastric tube in position

I. If patient chokes, cannot talk, or becomes cyanotic, tube is in trachea. Remove, allow patient to ventilate, and start again.

J. Tape tube to cheek. Avoid sharp bend at nostril which can produce irritation and later necrosis of the skin.

K. Keep patient sitting or semi-upright.

L. Apply suction to tube every 10 minutes. If no return, irrigate and ensure tube open with 5–10 ml normal saline or water.

Complications
A. Insertion into cranial vault in patients with cribriform plate fracture. Do not place in patients with suspected facial fractures.

B. Tracheal intubation.

C. Nasal trauma causing upper airway bleeding.

D. Vomiting and aspiration of gastric contents, either during insertion or while in place, particularly if stomach not decompressed.

Special Notes
A. Tube not indicated if transit time short or contraindications present.

B. There is little point in placing NG tube if it is allowed to clog or if no suction is applied. The tube overcomes the normal cardio-esophageal sphincter mechanism and allows reflux or regurgitation of stomach contents, so the patient must remain sitting or semi-upright.

C. Vigorous bleeding from stomach will quickly clog tube. Be ready to irrigate and aspirate frequently.

PNEUMATIC ANTI-SHOCK GARMENT (PASG) APPLICATION

Indications

A. Splinting major trauma to pelvis or lower extremities.

B. Blood pressure less than 90 mm Hg systolic AND signs of shock in a patient who has findings suggestive of hypovolemia. Physiologically may autotransfuse small quantities of blood but probably primary results are due to increased peripheral vascular resistance. Provides tamponade effect to slow bleeding in injuries below the diaphragm.

   1. Traumatic hypovolemia:

      a. Blunt or penetrating abdominal injury.

      b. Extremity fractures (especially femur) or amputations with major bleeding.

      c. Pelvis fractures.

   2. Non-traumatic hypovolemia:

      a. Upper or lower GI bleeding.

      b. Ruptured abdominal aneurysm.

      c. Vaginal or postpartum hemorrhage.

      d. Ruptured ectopic pregnancy.

C. Major trauma without hypotension (application without inflation) in anticipation of possibility of rapid deterioration.

D. Recent controversy has resulted in a variety of recommendations for use. Regional consensus should direct field care for any specific indications.

Precautions

A. One contraindication to inflation is pulmonary edema. If this occurs after suit is inflated, deflate abdominal section first, legs if needed.

B. *Not indicated with penetrating thoracic trauma.* This is probably the only situation that actually has data indicating patients do worse with the PASG being utilized.

C. Except in the presence of pulmonary edema, *do not deflate in the field*. Deflation is best managed in a hospital situation where IV lines are secure, blood is available and definitive intervention to stop bleeding can be started immediately.

D. Never inflate the abdominal section alone.

E. Although head injury may be aggravated by the fluid load of the PASG, altered consciousness can be caused by hypotension. Treatment for the hypotension takes precedence over head injury treatment. In a case of isolated head injury, discuss with base physician.

F. In visibly pregnant patients, avoid abdominal inflation.

G. Carefully note presence of wounds which the suit will cover once inflated.

H. Do not apply too low. Remember that the inflated chambers will shorten. The most common error is to apply so that the lower abdomen only is covered.

Technique

A. Obtain baseline vital signs.

B. Apply suit to backboard or stretcher prior to moving patient (Figure 7-28). Otherwise lift patient as unit and slide under.

C. Complete secondary survey. Document and briefly dress wounds which will be covered by suit.

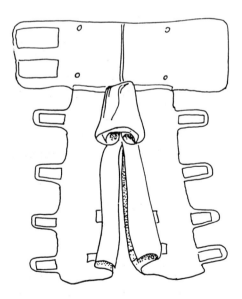

Figure 7-28. PASG

D. Apply PASG using Velcro straps. Legs first, then abdominal section if using single piece suit. Be sure abdominal section is positioned properly – to xiphoid, covering main abdominal surfaces (Figure 7-29).

E. Inflate with foot pump until patient improves (improved level of consciousness or BP > 90 mm Hg systolic). Stop when Velcro crackles or air exhausts through relief valves.

F. Close stopcock valves. If units are inflated separately, inflate leg units prior to abdominal unit.

G. Record time of inflation.

H. Listen to lungs and check for adequacy of ventilation.

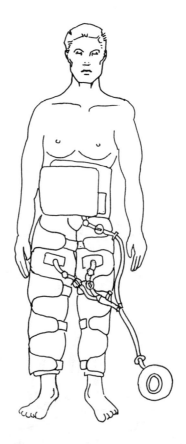

Figure 7-29. PASG in position

I. Recheck and record vital signs.

J. Monitor suit pressure and patient pressure en route and regulate inflation as needed.

Complications
A. Pulmonary edema from volume overload, particularly in elderly patients.

B. Ventilatory compromise from restriction of ribs if applied too high.

C. Inability to examine patient under suit. Inability to monitor skin color, temperature, circulation in lower extremities.

D. Vomiting, urination or defecation due to abdominal pressure at time of inflation.

E. Acidosis and circulatory compromise with long-term (over many hours) inflation.

Special Notes
A. Suit inflation may make IV line insertion easier in the hypovolemic patient.

B. Closed head injury is only a relative contraindication to the use of antishock suit. If hypovolemia is life-threatening, the suit is indicated. Try to stop bleeding before inflation. Benefits will be very transient in the presence of continued bleeding.

C. Use your patient's condition to monitor inflation. Minimal inflation can produce excellent results in some patients. Monitor the patient's pressure, *not* the suit pressure. Pedal pulses and capillary refill can still be monitored if suit pressure is not at maximum. Inflation pressure should only be as much as needed to stabilize patient.

D. Be familiar with deflation procedures and be willing to assist hospital personnel if needed.

E. Monitor inflation carefully. Leaks occur and adjustment is also needed during changes in altitude or temperature.

F. Do not inflate by blowing into tubes. You may find yourself with a mouthful of contamination.

G. The efficacy of the PASG is hotly debated. Its use has been abandoned in some systems. It is *never* a substitute for rapid transport for definitive care.

PERIPHERAL IV LINE INSERTION

Indications

A. Administer fluids for volume expansion.

B. Administer medications.

Precautions

Wear gloves and eye protection.

A. Do not start IVs distal to a fracture site or through skin damaged with more than erythema or superficial abrasion.

B. All IVs started in the field are considered contaminated and must be changed within 6 hours of insertion.

C. Make *certain* the IV solution prepared is the correct one.

D. If venous access is only required as a precaution or for drug administration, consider saline lock rather than risk inadvertent fluid administration.

Technique

A. Extremity

1. Explain the procedure to the patient.

2. Connect tubing to IV solution.

3. Fill drip chamber one-half full by squeezing (microdrip for cardiac patients or infants, macrodrip for trauma).

4. Tear sufficient tape to anchor IV in place.

5. Apply tourniquet proximal to proposed site, or use blood pressure cuff blown up to 40 mm Hg.

6. *Scrub* insertion site. (Betadine vs. alcohol is less important than vigor.)

7. Do not palpate, unless necessary, after prep. If you must palpate, prep your gloved finger.

8. Hold vein in place by applying gentle traction on vein distal to point of entry.

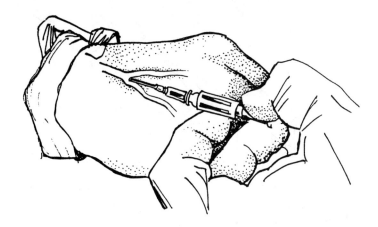

Figure 7-30. IV – peripheral

9. Puncture the skin with the bevel of the needle upward about 0.5 to 1 cm from the vein and enter the vein from the side or from above (Figure 7-30 and 7-31).

10. Note blood return and advance the catheter either over or through the needle (depending on type).

11. Remove needle and connect tubing. Note: blood for laboratory work may be drawn with syringe before connecting tubing. Assure proper disposal of "sharps".

12. Release tourniquet.

13. Open IV tubing clamp full to check flow and placement, then slow rate to TKO or as directed.

14. Cover puncture site with Betadine ointment on Band-Aid. Secure tubing with tape, making sure of at least one 180 degree turn in the tubing to be sure any traction on the tubing is not transmitted to the cannula itself. Label the tape indicating date, time, name of person starting the IV, and size of catheter or needle.

15. Anchor with arm board or splint as needed to minimize chance of losing line with movement.

16. *Recheck* to be sure IV rate is as desired, and monitor.

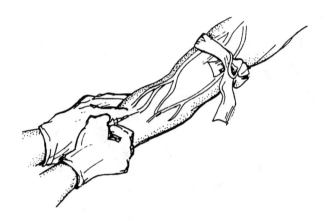

Figure 7-31. IV antecubital

B. External jugular vein (Figure 7-32 and 7-33)

   1. Explain the procedure to the patient.

   2. Connect tubing to IV solution.

   3. Fill drip chamber one-half full by squeezing (microdrip for cardiac patients or infants, macrodrip for trauma).

   4. Tear sufficient tape to anchor IV in place.

   5. Position the patient – supine, head down (this may not be necessary or desirable if congestive heart failure or respiratory distress present). Turn patient's head to opposite side from procedure.

   6. Expose vein by having patient bear down if possible, and "tourniquet" vein with finger pressure just above clavicle.

   7. *Scrub* insertion site. (Betadine vs. alcohol is less important than vigor.)

   8. Do not palpate, unless necessary, after prep. If you must palpate, prep your gloved finger.

   9. Align the cannula in the direction of the vein, with the point aimed toward the shoulder on the same side.

   10. Puncture skin over vein first, then puncture vein itself. Use other hand to traction vein near clavicle to prevent rolling.

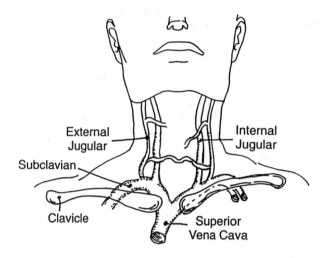

Figure 7-32. External jugular vein

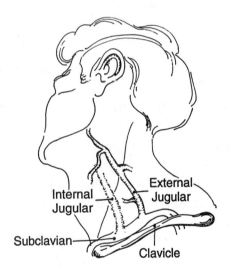

Figure 7-33. External jugular – lateral view

11. Attach syringe and aspirate if pressure in vein not sufficient to give flash-back. Advance cannula well into vein once it is penetrated. Attach IV tubing. Assure proper disposal of "sharps".

12. Open IV tubing clamp full to check flow and placement, then slow rate to TKO or as directed.

13. Cover puncture site with Betadine ointment on Band-Aid. Secure tubing with tape, making sure of at least one 180 degree turn in the tubing to be sure any traction on the tubing is not transmitted to the cannula itself. Label the tape indicating date, time, name of person starting the IV, and size of catheter or needle.

14. *Recheck* to be sure IV rate is as desired, and monitor.

C. Scalp Vein – *For use by physician order in pediatric patients* (Usually less than 1 year of age)

1. Connect tubing to IV solution RL.

2. Fill microdrip chamber one-half full by squeezing.

3. Tear sufficient tape to secure butterfly once in place.

4. Select a 23–25 gauge butterfly and a 1–2 ml syringe filled with 1 ml saline.

5. Place large rubber band or tourniquet around the infant's head above the ears and across top of forehead.

6. Locate vessel. (Frequently just anterior and superior to ear.)

7. Shave an area large enough to not only expose the vessel(s) but to allow for adequate taping.

8. Palpate the vessel to assure that it is venous and has no pulsations.

9. *Scrub* insertion site. (Betadine vs. alcohol is less important than vigor.)

10. Puncture the skin approximately 0.5 cm from the vessel to be cannulated and aim in the direction of blood flow (usually toward the neck or face).

11. Ensure free flow of blood, then attach syringe, release the tourniquet and inject slowly 0.5 ml of saline. If the needle is in good position the solution will flow readily. The syringe may then be replaced with IV tubing. If the needle has dislodged, a wheal will indicate poor placement and another site must be chosen. Assure proper disposal of "sharps".

12. Cover puncture site with Betadine ointment and tape securely. Cotton balls or gauze may be needed to support hub to keep needle in line with vein for free flow.

13. Tape additional loop of tubing at a distance to absorb any tension.

14. *Recheck* to be sure IV rate is as desired, and monitor.

D. Saline Lock

1. Explain the procedure to the patient.

2. Tear sufficient tape to anchor lock in place.

3. Select an appropriate sized catheter and fill a 10 ml syringe with 10 ml saline.

4. Apply tourniquet proximal to proposed site, or use blood pressure cuff blown up to 40 mm Hg.

5. *Scrub* insertion site. (Betadine vs. alcohol is less important than vigor.)

6. Do not palpate, unless necessary, after prep. If you must palpate, prep your gloved finger.

7. Hold vein in place by applying gentle traction on vein distal to point of entry.

8. Puncture the skin with the bevel of the needle upward about 0.5 to 1 cm from the vein and enter the vein from the side or from above.

9. Note blood return and advance the catheter either over or through the needle (depending on type). Assure proper disposal of "sharps".

10. Release tourniquet.

11. Flush catheter with 10 ml saline to assure good position.

12. Cover puncture site with Betadine ointment on Band-Aid. Label the tape indicating date, time, name of person starting the lock, and size of catheter or needle.

Complications

A. Pyogenic reactions due to contaminated fluids become evident in about 30 minutes after starting the IV. Patient will develop fever, chills, nausea, vomiting, headache, or general malaise. If observed, stop and remove IV immediately. Save the solution so it may be cultured.

B. Local – hematoma formation, infection, thrombosis, phlebitis. Note: The incidence of phlebitis is particularly high in the leg. Avoid use of lower extremity if possible.

C. Systemic – sepsis, catheter fragment embolus, or fiber embolus from IV solution.

Special Notes
A. Antecubital veins are useful access sites for patients in shock, but otherwise, avoid areas near joints (or splint well!).

B. The point between the junction of two veins is more stable and often easier to use.

C. Start distally, and if successive attempts are necessary, you will be able to make more proximal attempts on the same vein without extravasating IV fluid.

D. In difficult situations, do not forget "butterflies". They are often easier and may be better than no line at all.

E. Venipuncture itself is seldom morbid. The excess fluids inadvertently run in when nobody is watching can be fatal!

F. The most difficult problem with IV insertion is to know when to try and when to stop trying. Valuable time is often wasted attempting IVs when a critical patient requires blood. IV solutions may "buy time", but they frequently lose time instead. Generally, one attempt at the scene may be worthwhile, other attempts should be en route.

G. Saline locks are becoming increasingly popular in the world of "cost containment". The use also allows a patient to be unencumbered by trailing IV lines. This may be particularly useful in situations where there is an awkward extrication (narrow hallways and stairs) and inclement weather where fluid can freeze in IV line while loading. The greatest risk is establishing an inadequate line that is unrecognized. The saline flush of 10 ml should usually be sufficient to detect a line that is not patent, but don't hesitate to add additional fluid if necessary to detect a subcutaneous or inadequate catheterization.

RESTRAINT

Indications

A. A patient who needs to be transported for medical care, who is refusing transport or care, *and* who is incompetent to refuse.

B. A person who appears to be mentally ill and who, as a result of such mental illness, appears to be an imminent danger to others or to himself *or* to be gravely disabled.

C. Physician consult by phone or radio which confirms above judgments.

Precautions

A. Any attempt at restraint involves risk to patient and EMT or Paramedic. Do not attempt to restrain a patient without adequate assistance.

B. Physical restraints are a last resort. All possible means of verbal persuasion should be attempted first.

C. A patient who is alert, oriented, aware of his condition, and capable of understanding the consequences of his refusal is entitled to refuse treatment. He may not be restrained and treated against his will. (Review consent guidelines and confer with physician if in doubt.)

D. If there is a significant chance of the patient vomiting (e.g., intoxicants, withdrawal states), do not restrain in supine position, but rather in lateral position to decrease risk of aspiration.

Techniques

A. Determine that patient's medical or mental condition requires ambulance transport to the emergency department *and* that patient lacks decision-making capacity, *or* that there is a basis for police or mental health hold.

B. Obtain adequate manpower for assistance.

C. Treat the patient with respect.

D. Organize your help in advance. Assign at least one person to each limb. A fifth person can coordinate the procedure.

E. Have all equipment ready.

F. Equipment must be durable and in good condition to avoid tearing or breaking with resultant injury to patient or rescuers.

G. Inform the patient of your need to restrain him. Explain the procedure to the patient.

H. Restrain arms and legs. Avoid body restraints as they may result in strangulation.

I. Reassure patient, remind him that you are there to assist him in getting care.

J. Check restraints as soon as applied and every 10 minutes thereafter to ensure no injury to extremities.

K. Pad restraints as necessary.

L. Paper face masks or oxygen masks (with adequate oxygen/air supply) may be useful to control spitting or biting. Tape mask over nose and mouth.

M. Once in restraints – do not leave the patient at any time.

N. Remove restrains only with sufficient personnel available to control patient – generally, only in the hospital.

O. Document indication for restraints, type of restraints, monitoring during transport, and condition on arrival at emergency department.

Complications

A. Radial nerve palsy (sensory loss on hand) can result from pinching of the nerve by hard restraints over the wrist prominences.

B. Aspiration can occur if patient is restrained on his back and cannot protect his own airway.

C. Medical causes for combativeness, if overlooked, may result in further injury to patient or inappropriate placement. Do not forget the medical differential of altered mental states – hypoglycemia, hypoxia, stroke, hyperthermia, hypothermia, or drug ingestion.

D. Deterioration may cause your patient to "calm down". Be sure you are not falsely reassured.

Special Notes

A. Use with caution in patients with extremity injuries.

B. Written and verbal reports must completely document the necessity for the use of physical restraints.

SPLINTING: AXIAL

Indications
A. Pain, swelling or deformity of spine which may be due to fracture, dislocation, or ligamentous instability.

B. Neurologic deficit which might be due to spine injury.

C. Prevention of neurologic deficit or further deficit in patients with suspected spine injury or instability.

D. In all trauma victims who are unconscious or with impaired consciousness due to head injury or drug ingestion, to protect against damage or further damage in patients where injury to the spine cannot be ruled out by accurate exam or history.

Precautions
A. All patients with significant head trauma should be immobilized because of the potential for unrecognized coexistent neck trauma.

B. Perform and document complete neurologic exam prior to movement if at all possible. Redocument after your splinting is complete.

Cervical Splinting Technique
A. Apply following primary assessment if indicated. Use assistant to maintain cervical stabilization while completing primary survey.

B. Use two persons to apply splint if at all possible.

C. Have assistant apply gentle continuous traction in neutral axis of spine. Do not use force to straighten.

D. Advise patient of procedure and purpose before and during application.

E. Immobilize the cervical spine with a semi-rigid or rigid Philadelphia collar.

F. Use long spine board, short board or KED (or similar device) to support patient as situation dictates.

G. Pad behind head in adults to maintain anatomically neutral position (Figure 7-34). Pad under the torso to maintain anatomically neutral position in children (Figure 7-35).

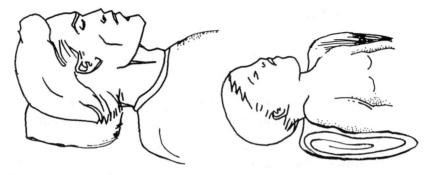

Figure 7-34. Padding, adult   **Figure 7-35.** Padding, child

H. Use tape, straps, or both to secure patient effectively and allow turning as a unit for airway control. Secure torso first, then head and neck, extremities last.

I. Request assistant to monitor airway and security of immobilization.

Spine Immobilization Technique

A. Splint cervical spine with rigid collar following primary survey.

B. Complete secondary survey and splint fractures prior to movement of patient when possible.

C. Document neurologic findings.

D. In a sitting patient, use short board, KED, or similar device for extrication:

   1. Slide short board, if needed, behind patient.

   2. Apply thigh straps snugly as close to groin as possible.

   3. Apply shoulder straps.

   4. Use padding as needed to keep neck in cervical collar in a neutral position.

   5. Secure head to board with tape or cloths.

E. Use long board for supine patients or sitting patients after short board, KED or similar device applied (Figure 7-36):

   1. Apply PASG to board, if needed, before moving patient.

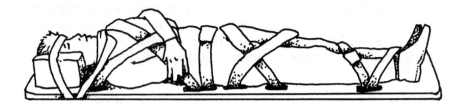

Figure 7-36. Spinal immobilization

2. Logroll or lift patient as a unit to board. Apply continuous cervical stabilization during movement. One person should protect neck in collar. Do not use force to straighten spine.

3. Release leg straps if short board, KED, or similar device used.

4. Use padding as needed behind knees to support a neutral axis under small of back, neck and knees.

5. Secure trunk to long spine board.

6. Pad behind the head as needed to maintain anatomically neutral position, pad under torso for pediatric patients.

7. Use sandbags, rolls, or blocks and tape to secure neck.

8. Apply straps or tape to secure thighs, and lower legs to allow turning as a unit in case of vomiting or airway difficulty.

F. Reassess patient status, particularly airway and neurologic findings.

G. Assign assistant to monitor airway and neck immobilization.

Complications

A. Vomiting is common in head/spine injured patients. Your splinting must be good enough to allow turning of the patient for airway protection.

B. Cord injury with neurologic deficit may be accompanied by neurogenic shock. Elevate foot of long board 10–12" or prop legs on blankets and secure with tape. Watch also for the more dangerous hypovolemia!

C. It is easy to miss injuries below the level of a neurological deficit. Look carefully for abdominal and chest injuries, pelvis fractures, and extremity injuries without symptoms. With an injury and loss of sensation below T-8, there will be no guarding, rebound, or tenderness to clue you to internal abdominal injuries.

Special Notes

A. Pelvis fractures are difficult to diagnose in the field. Suspected pelvis injury can be immobilized by use of the long board during spine immobilization. Grossly unstable fractures could be stabilized and tamponaded with the PASG.

B. It is the patient without neurologic deficit, or with only partial deficit, who most needs your care and protection from further injury.

C. While the concern needs to be high and the decision to immobilize needs to be liberal, there are a significant number of patients who have been in accidents, are alert, oriented, *not* intoxicated – who have no neck pain and no tenderness. These patients *do not* need to be immobilized due to "mechanism of injury". That only applies to patients who are not able to adequately evaluate their environment – whether due to alcohol, hypoxia, or head injury.

D. Spinal immobilization *at its best* is uncomfortable. Studies have shown that immobilization on a firm spine board *causes* back and neck pain. Immobilize appropriately, pad liberally, and explain to the patients the need for this procedure. Many patients dislike being "strapped" down and tolerate the procedure better when advised they are being "belted in" with "seat belts".

SPLINTING: EXTREMITY

Indications

A. Pain, swelling or deformity in extremity which may be due to fracture or dislocation.

B. In an unstable extremity injury – to reduce pain, limit bleeding at the site of injury, and prevent further injury to soft tissues, blood vessels or nerves.

Precautions

A. Critically injured trauma victims should not be delayed in transport by lengthy evaluation of possible noncritical extremity injuries. Prevention of further damage may be accomplished by securing the patient to a spine board when other injuries demand prompt hospital treatment.

B. The patient with altered level of consciousness from head injury or drug influences should be carefully examined and conservatively treated because his ability to recognize pain and injury is impaired.

C. Make sure the obvious injury is also the only one. It is particularly easy to miss fractures proximal to the most visible one.

D. In a stable patient in which no environmental hazard exists, splinting should be done prior to moving the patient.

E. Never deliberately test for crepitus or instability.

F. Air splints are useful to control bleeding, but avoid overinflation and circulatory compromise. Temperature and altitude changes during transport will alter splint pressure.

Extremity Splinting Technique

A. Check pulse and sensation distally prior to movement.

B. Remove bracelets, watches, or other constricting bands prior to splint application. (Tape objects to patients.)

C. Identify and dress open wounds. Note wounds which contain exposed bone or lie near fracture sites and may communicate with a fracture.

D. Avoid unnecessary movement of fracture site to minimize pain and soft tissue damage.

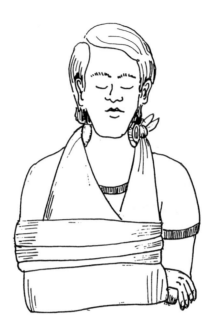

Figure 7-37. Sling and swathe

E. Choose splint to immobilize joint above and below injury (Figure 7-37). Pad rigid splints to prevent pressure injury to extremity.

F. Apply gentle continuous traction to extremity and support to fracture site during splinting operation.

G. Reduce angulated fractures, including open fractures, with gentle axial traction as needed to immobilize properly.

H. Check distal pulses and sensation after reduction and splinting. Remanipulate gently or replace in original position if adequate circulation and sensation is lost.

Traction Splinting Technique (for suspected femur fractures only) (Figure 7-38)

A. Use two persons for splint application procedure.

B. Remove sock and shoe and check for distal pulse and sensation (unless you cannot protect exposed foot from weather, then just ask patient about sensation and observe movement).

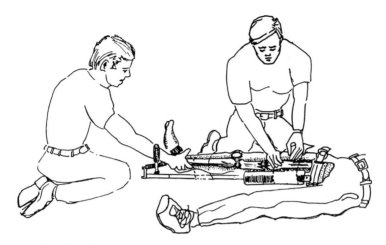

Figure 7-38. Traction splinting

C. Identify and dress open wounds and note exposed bone or wounds overlying fractures as potential communicating wounds.

D. Measure splint length prior to application.

E. Apply gentle axial traction with support to calf and fracture site, reducing angulation or open fractures as necessary for secure traction splinting.

F. Position ischial pad under buttocks up against bony prominence (ischial tuberosity). Empty pockets if needed.

G. Secure groin strap. Carefully!

H. Maintain continuous traction and support to fracture site throughout procedure.

I. Adjust support straps to appropriate positions under leg.

J. Apply ankle hitch and tighten traction until patient experiences improved comfort. (Movement at the fracture site will cause some pain, but if traction continues to cause increased pain, do not proceed. Splint and support leg in position of most comfort.)

K. Secure support straps after traction properly adjusted.

L. Recheck distal pulses and sensation.

M. Apply PASG over traction splint if indicated.

Complications

A. Circulatory compromise from excessive constriction of limb.

B. Continued bleeding not visible under splint.

C. Pressure damage to skin and nerves from inadequate padding.

D. Delayed treatment of life-threatening injuries due to prolonged splinting procedures.

Special Notes

A. Traction splints should only be used if the leg can be straightened easily and patient is comfortable with the traction device in place. Particularly with injuries about the hip and knee, forced application of traction device can cause increased pain and damage. If this occurs, do not use traction device but support leg with pillows, sandbags, or other support in position of most comfort and best neurovascular status.

B. Traction technique described is most specific for Hare traction device. There are several devices available and slight modifications in application technique are needed. The principles should remain the same, however. It is always essential to become knowledgeable about your own equipment.

C. When in doubt and patient stable, splint. Do not be deceived by absence of deformity or disability. Fractured limbs often retain some ability to function.

D. PASG can be used effectively as a long-leg air splint or to stabilize pelvis fractures. PASG is probably a much more appropriate splint for the multiple trauma patient who also has a femur fracture. Traction splinting is most appropriate for the isolated femur fracture.

E. Splinting body parts together can be a very effective way of immobilizing (e.g., arm-to-trunk or leg-to-leg). Padding will increase comfort. This method can be very useful in children when traction devices and premade splints do not fit.

TENSION PNEUMOTHORAX DECOMPRESSION

Philosophy

Tension pneumothorax is not only rare, it is an extremely difficult diagnosis to make in the field with any accuracy. The physical examination of the chest is notoriously unreliable in the freshly traumatized chest and the patient with chronic obstructive lung disease may well have dyspnea at rest, cyanosis, and absent breath sounds unilaterally or bilaterally without having even a simple pneumothorax, no less a tension pneumothorax. Probably the most helpful diagnostic sign is rapidly increasing air hunger in a cyanotic patient who has a history compatible with pneumothorax (e.g., someone kicked in the chest). The most common use of the procedure in the field is in the traumatized patient who has been intubated and rapidly becomes increasingly difficult to bag. This patient will need decompression immediately. This skill (diagnosis *and* technique) must be reviewed and practiced if it is to be ready on the rare occasion when it is indicated.

Indications

A. Patient with pneumothorax (Figure 7-39) who requires air transport (with altitude changes).

B. *Increasing* respiratory insufficiency in a susceptible patient:

   1. Untreated spontaneous pneumothorax.

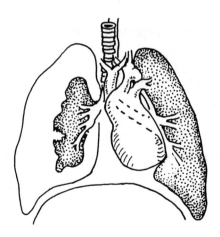

Figure 7-39. Pneumothorax

2. CPR with PEA, increased difficulty bagging patient.

3. Sucking chest wound which has been covered completely.

4. Chest trauma with suspected pneumothorax.

Precautions
Wear gloves and eye protection.

A. Classic physical findings are often not present. You must be suspicious in patients who may be susceptible. This is a rare but life-threatening diagnosis.

B. Recognize the difference between the two types of pneumothorax:

Simple pneumothorax

1. Respiratory distress (mild to severe).

2. Chest pain.

3. *May* have decreased or absent breath sounds on the side of the collapse (not necessarily!)

4. Subcutaneous air if the cause is traumatic.

Tension pneumothorax

1. Progressive respiratory distress.

2. Dropping BP.

3. "Drum-like" hyperexpanded chest.

4. Distended neck veins.

5. General patient deterioration.

6. If intubated, progressive difficulty in bagging.

Tracheal shift is rarely present.

C. Pneumothorax rarely presents with tension on the initial assessment. Be particularly suspicious with deterioration during transport and with patients requiring assisted ventilation.

Technique
A. Direct physician communication must be made for approval to treat if time is available.

B. If covered sucking chest wound is present, remove the seal and allow chest pressures to equilibrate. May need no further treatment.

C. Needle decompression (angiocath only) (Figure 7-40)

1. Expose the entire chest.

2. Clean area for insertion vigorously – alcohol or Betadine.

3. Attach 20 ml syringe or leave angiocath open.

4. Insert angiocath into the pleural space by entering the chest in the second or third intercostal space in the mid-clavicular line. The catheter should be inserted on top of the rib so as to avoid the intercostal vessels and nerves which run below each rib.

5. When tension is present, plunger will back out of syringe or an immediate hiss of air escaping will be heard. Some of the newer catheters will not allow air passage until the needle is withdrawn and the plastic hub as the only part remaining allows the air to escape. If there is no initial hiss – remove the needle and reevaluate. A second catheter may be needed with severe air leak.

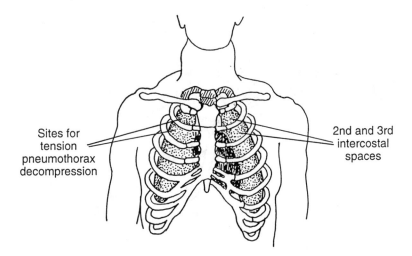

Sites for tension pneumothorax decompression

2nd and 3rd intercostal spaces

Figure 7-40. Needle decompression of tension pneumothorax

6. If no hiss or evidence of tension seen, remove angiocath and reassess reason for patient deterioration.

7. If air under pressure is demonstrated, remove the needle trocar and advance the catheter.

8. Tape in place.

9. Connect to flutter valve if available (Figure 7-41). Otherwise, simply ventilate the patient.

D. If patient deteriorates after needle decompression, be prepared to assist ventilation and continue hyper-oxygenating.

Complications
A. Creation of pneumothorax if none existed previously.

B. Pulmonary edema from release of collapsed lung, particularly in spontaneous pneumothorax.

C. Laceration of lung.

D. Laceration of blood vessels – slide *above* rib (intercostal vessels run in groove under each rib).

E. Infection – clean rapidly but vigorously, use sterile gloves if possible.

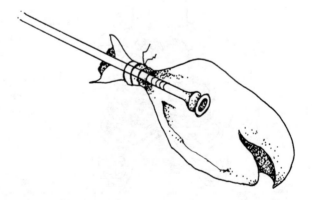

Figure 7-41. Flutter valve

Special Notes

A. The procedure is very painful. It should never be performed unless the patient is in extremis. It is impossible to completely deaden the pleura. Rapid penetration of the pleura will be kindest for the patient.

B. Sudden onset of chest pain and shortness of breath in a normal individual may be caused by a pneumothorax. These can also progress to a "tension" state, but rarely do so. The differential for respiratory distress, particularly in the COPD patient, is long. Field diagnosis is difficult. And the addition of a pneumothorax by inappropriate diagnosis can be fatal. Unless the patient is intubated with positive pressure ventilation, procedure should not be attempted.

C. In CPR with PEA and possible tension pneumothorax, decompress both sides of chest (*after* intubation).

D. Although tension pneumothorax decompression is a hazardous procedure and has been listed as *direct physician order*, it is apparent that in circumstances where this technique is actually essential for the patient's breathing – there may be no time to make a phone/radio call. In those "time critical" instances, it is better to perform the needed procedure, then document the circumstances in an incident report.

8

PREHOSPITAL MEDICATIONS

INTRODUCTION TO PREHOSPITAL DRUGS

These drugs are listed in alphabetical order. Both basic and advanced medications are included. Not all medications are appropriate for all systems.

Basic prehospital drugs:

    Dextrose, oral preparations
    Oxygen
    Charcoal
    Assist patient with – epinephrine (Epi-Pen) or anaphylaxis kit
    inhalers and nitroglycerin

Advanced drugs suitable for standing-order *or* direct-order administration

    Albuterol
    Atropine
    Bretylium
    Charcoal
    Dextrose, IV preparations
    Diphenhydramine
    Epinephrine (cardiac arrest)

IV solutions
Lidocaine
Naloxone
Nitroglycerin
Phenylephrine nasal spray
Sodium bicarbonate (drowning, cardiac arrest)

Advanced drugs to be administered only by direct order:

Adenosine
Calcium
Diazepam
Dopamine
Droperidol
Epinephrine (anaphylaxis, asthma)
Furosemide
Glucagon
Ipecac
Magnesium sulfate
Morphine
Oxytocin
Racemic epinephrine
Verapamil

ADENOSINE (ADENOCARD)

Pharmacology and actions
Adenosine is a naturally occurring purine nucleoside found in all body cells. Adenosine slows conduction time through the AV node. This results in an interruption of AV-nodal reentry pathways. It often restores NSR in patients with PSVT.

Indications
A. PSVT (Including PSVT associated with Wolff-Parkinson-White Syndrome or other accessory bypass tracts.)

B. Tachycardia of uncertain etiology, to assist with determination of underlying dysrhythmia.

Precautions
A. Contraindicated in patients with second or third degree A-V block or sick sinus syndrome unless they have an adequately functioning pacemaker. Underlying blocks or conduction defects can be associated with prolonged sinus arrest or AV blocks when using adenosine.

B. Adenosine has a very short half-life (< 10 seconds). If bolus administration is not rapid, followed by a fluid push, the drug may have no effect, simply because it has been metabolized.

C. The effects of adenosine are antagonized by methylxanthines (caffeine or theophyllines). Large doses of adenosine may be necessary, or the drug may not be effective in patients who are on high doses of theophyllines (such as asthmatics).

Administration – by direct physician order only.

Adults

Initial dose – 6 mg rapid IV push, followed immediately by a saline flush of 10–20 ml.

Second dose, if necessary after 1–2 minutes– 12 mg rapid IV push followed by saline flush. This may be repeated once if necessary.

Pediatrics

Initial dose – 0.1 mg/kg rapid IV push, followed immediately by a 3–5 ml saline flush.

Second dose, if necessary after 1–2 minutes – 0.2 mg/kg rapid IV push, followed by saline flush.

Side effects and special notes

A. At the time of conversion many patients will experience flushing, dyspnea, chest pain, or apprehension. These symptoms are usually very transient, but can be frightening to the patient. Reassurance will be helpful, particularly if given in advance.

B. The cardiac rhythm after administration of adenosine can undergo various dysrhythmias prior to converting to sinus rhythm. A brief period of asystole, bradycardia or transient ectopy is common.

ALBUTEROL

Pharmacology and actions
Albuterol is a relatively selective Beta$_2$ adrenergic stimulator. The effects are predominantly on bronchial smooth muscle, however there are also β_2 receptors in the heart muscle. Clinical effects most frequently include:

A. Bronchial dilatation, with improvement in FEV1 and peak flow rate within 5 minutes.

B. Tachycardia.

C. Peripheral vasodilatation.

D. Hyper- or hypotension possible.

Indications
Albuterol is indicated as a bronchodilator for asthma, and for reversible bronchospasm associated with bronchitis and emphysema (COPD).

Precautions
A. Use with caution in patients who have a history of cardiovascular disorders such as hypertension, coronary artery disease, congestive heart failure, or hyperthyroidism.

B. May lower seizure threshold in susceptible patients.

C. Patients over 40 should have cardiac rhythm monitored during treatment.

D. Paradoxical bronchospasm has been reported as a response to this drug. Whether that is actually a response or simply the underlying disease is difficult to determine. If it appears the patient is getting worse – discontinue the treatment and contact base physician.

Administration
A. Available as premixed solution 0.083% albuterol or 0.83 mg/ml or 2.5 mg/inhalation treatment.

B. *Adults* – administer by nebulizer 3 ml (2.5 mg for 2 yrs to adult).

   For infants or children under 2 – use half of the premixed solution; add 2 ml of saline.

C. May repeat or even administer as a continuous nebulization during transport if necessary.

Side effects and special notes

A. Nervousness, tremors, tachycardia and nausea are the most frequent side effects.

B. Occasionally may produce hypertension, palpitations, angina, or dysrhythmias.

C. Cardiac effects may be more pronounced in patients who are taking MAO inhibitors or tricyclic antidepressants.

D. Basic prehospital care providers may be asked to assist with administration of the patient's inhaler. Contact base physician to assess the type of inhaler and whether appropriate for current condition.

ATROPINE

Pharmacology and actions
Atropine is a parasympathetic or cholinergic blocking agent. As such, it has the following effects:

A. Increases heart rate (by blocking vagal influences).

B. Increases conduction through A-V node.

C. Reduces motility and tone of GI tract.

D. Reduces action and tone of urinary bladder (may cause urinary retention).

E. Dilates pupils.

Note: This drug blocks cholinergic (vagal) influences already present. If there is little cholinergic stimulation present, effects will be minimal.

Indications
A. To counteract excessive vagal influences responsible for some bradysystolic and asystolic arrests.

B. To increase heart rate in hemodynamically significant bradycardias.

C. To improve conduction in 2nd and 3rd degree heart block or in pacemaker failure.

D. As an antidote for some insecticide exposures (e.g., organophosphates) and nerve gases with symptoms of excess cholinergic stimulation: salivation, constricted pupils. bradycardia, tearing, diaphoresis, vomiting, and diarrhea.

Precautions
A. Bradycardias in the setting of an acute MI are common and may be beneficial. Do not treat them unless there are signs of poor perfusion (low blood pressure, mental confusion). Chest pain could be due to an MI or to poor perfusion caused by the bradycardia itself. When in doubt, consult the base physician.

B. People do well with chronic 2nd and 3rd degree block. Symptoms occur mainly with acute change. *Treat the patient, not the rhythm.*

C. Pediatric bradycardias are most commonly secondary to hypoxia.

283

Correct the ventilation first and treat the rate directly only if improved ventilation does not increase the rate.

D. Bradycardia in the trauma patient, as with the pediatric patient, is usually a result of underlying condition. It may be secondary to a cardiac contusion, or may be due to critical CNS, cardiac or respiratory decompensation. Treat the underlying cause!

Administration
A. Asystole

adult – 1.0 mg IV, repeat in 3–5 minutes to total of 0.04 mg/kg.

pediatric – 0.02 mg/kg per dose IV (minimum dose of 0.1 mg and a Max of 1.0 mg in child, Max of 2.0 mg in an adolescent).

B. Symptomatic bradycardia

adult – 0.5–1.0 mg IV, repeated if needed at 5 minute intervals to a heart rate of 60 or total of 0.04 mg/kg.

pediatric – 0.02 mg/kg per dose IV.

C. May be given via ET tube at double the dose.

D. For symptomatic insecticide exposures: contact base or PCC for dosage (usually begin with 2 mg IV and titrate). Total required dose may be massive.

Side effects and special notes
A. Remember in cardiac arrest situation that atropine dilates pupils.

B. Atropine should not be administered in less than 0.5 mg dose for adults to prevent a parasympathomimetic response that would further slow the heart rate.

BRETYLIUM

Pharmacology and actions
Bretylium is an adrenergic blocking drug that directly increases the ventricular fibrillation threshold in the heart. It also makes repolarization in normal and ischemic myocardium more uniform, thus decreasing the likelihood of re-entrant rhythms. Effects on adrenergic receptors in the heart cause an immediate transient rise of blood pressure following administration (occasionally increased heart rate and ventricular irritability are also seen). This is followed by adrenergic blockade, which causes hypotension (usually mild but sometimes significant). Bretylium has a different mechanism of action than other antidysrhythmics and does not depress contractility or conduction. Chemical defibrillation (conversion of ventricular fibrillation to an organized rhythm) has been reported after rapid IV bretylium without electrical defibrillation.

Indications
A. Ventricular fibrillation unresponsive to lidocaine, electrical countershock or epinephrine.

B. Ventricular tachycardia unresponsive to lidocaine.

C. Serious ectopic ventricular dysrhythmias unresponsive to lidocaine.

Precautions
Rapid IV administration should not be used in the awake patient because nausea and vomiting often occur.

Administration
A. In ventricular fibrillation or severe ventricular tachycardia –5 mg/ kg rapid IV (usual *adult dose* – 300–400 mg). Flush with 20 ml saline bolus and defibrillate. If no effect, give 10 mg/kg and repeat twice at 5–30 minute intervals if needed. Maximum dose 35 mg/ kg. *Pediatric dose* is the same – 5 mg/kg IV, repeat at 10 mg/kg IV.

B. In awake patient – dilute 5–10 mg/kg in 50 ml D5W or NS and give IV over 10 minutes.

C. One ampule = 10 ml = 500 mg.

Side effects and special notes

A. Hypotension due to adrenergic blockade is the most common side effect. Leg elevation and fluids will usually reverse this. Pressor agents are rarely needed.

B. Because bretylium works by a different mechanism than lidocaine, the two may be complementary and produce a synergistic response. The relative value of each in intractable ventricular fibrillation is still a matter of study and debate.

CALCIUM

Pharmacology and actions
A. Increases contractility of cardiac muscle.

B. May increase ventricular automaticity and excitability.

C. Decreases heart rate.

D. Produces effects similar to and additive with those of digitalis.

Indications
A. Hypocalcemia.

B. Hyperkalemia.

C. Hypermagnesemia.

D. Calcium channel blocker toxicity.

Precautions
A. Do not add to IV in rapid succession with sodium bicarbonate (precipitates calcium salt).

B. In digitalized patients, additive effects may cause ventricular fibrillation or asystole.

Administration – by direct physician order only.
A. Calcium chloride (10% solution) 1 ampule or prefilled syringe = 10 ml = 13.6 mEq calcium = 1000 mg calcium chloride.

B. *Adult dose* – 10 mg/kg calcium chloride slow IV (7 ml 10% solution for 70 kg patient).

C. *Pediatric dose* – 20 mg/kg calcium chloride (0.2 ml/kg) slow IV to a maximum of 2 ml.

Side effects and special notes
A. If heart is beating, rapid administration of calcium salts can produce bradycardia or asystole.

B. May increase cardiac irritability (PVCs), particularly in the presence of digitalis.

C. Local infiltration into the subcutaneous tissue will cause tissue necrosis. Be sure the IV is secure.

CHARCOAL

Pharmacology and actions
Oral activated charcoal adsorbs drugs and chemicals on the surface of the charcoal particles. This adsorption is almost irreversible and prevents absorption and toxicity. Activated charcoal is produced by the destruction of various organic materials (wood, petroleum) then treated at high temperature with activating agents (steam or CO_2) to increase its adsorptive capacity. Activation occurs by removing previously adsorbed materials and by reducing particle size, thereby increasing the surface area.

Indications
A. Toxic ingestion of chemicals (other than acids, alkalis or hydrocarbons).

B. Overdose of medications (other than iron or lithium).

Precautions
A. Do not administer soon after ipecac since it may come up rather violently. It is very difficult to clean from clothing and surroundings.

B. If administering via NG tube – assure that the tube is in the stomach. Charcoal is not helpful to the lungs.

C. Do not administer to comatose patient; ABCs will take precedence in those patients.

Administration – by direct physician or Poison Control Center (PCC) order.

A. *Adult* – 1 gm/kg activated charcoal orally or via NG tube.

B. *Pediatric* – 1 gm/kg orally.

Side effects and special notes
A. Charcoal is inert with very few side effects, but may be constipating.

B. Charcoal is useful in many ingestions. It is most effective when administered soon after the ingestion, but may still be effective many hours later.

C. There are some ingestions that are not adsorbed by charcoal (iron, lithium, alcohols, caustics). Contact base physician to discuss specific ingestions. Order for administration may also come from PCC if family has been in communication with them or PCC easier to contact.

D. Basic prehospital care providers may administer with direct physician order.

DEXTROSE

Pharmacology and actions
Glucose is the body's basic fuel. It produces most of the body's quick energy. Glucose use is regulated by insulin, which stimulates storage of excess glucose from the bloodstream, and by glucagon, which mobilizes stored glucose in the bloodstream.

Indications
A. Any illness or altered mental state in a known diabetic which might be caused by hypoglycemia.

B. Unconscious patient when a history is unobtainable and hypoglycemia cannot be excluded.

C. In patients with any focal neurologic deficit or altered state of consciousness and a blood glucose < 60 mg/dl.

D. Patient with active seizure or cardiac arrest when history is unobtainable.

E. Pediatric patients (less than 3) with signs of shock.

F. Hypothermia, generalized.

G. Any clinical condition of concern for hypoglycemia and blood glucose reading less than 60 mg/dl.

Precautions
A. Draw one red top tube or test 1–2 drops of blood prior to administration of dextrose.

B. Extravasation of dextrose will cause necrosis of tissue. IV should be secure and free return of blood into the syringe or tubing should be checked 2–3 times during administration.

Administration
A. Draw one red top tube (5 ml) of blood, or test blood for glucose level.

B. *Adult* – 50 ml ampule 50% dextrose (1 ml/kg) IV into secure vein if patient unable to tolerate oral fluids.

C. *Pediatric* – 2 ml/kg 25% dextrose (dilute 50:50 with saline) into secure IV.

D. *Neonates* – 5 ml/kg of *10%* dextrose (dilute 1:5 with saline) into secure IV.

E. Give 50% dextrose solution orally (or sugar plus juice, honey, molasses, syrup) if patient is awake.

Side effects and special notes

A. Dextrose is remarkably free of side effects for most patients and should be used whenever a question of hypoglycemia exists.

B. In an unconscious patient, blood should be drawn for glucose determination and a drop should be tested. If results are low or equivocal, administer dextrose. Dextrose should be omitted only with a clear cut test reading over 100 mg/dl.

C. Effect is delayed in elderly people with poor circulation or patients who have been hypoglycemic for a prolonged period of time.

D. Do not draw blood for glucose determination from site proximal to an IV containing glucose or dextrose.

E. There are some patients who do not need (and may even be made worse) by the administration of IV dextrose. This is particularly true of the older patients with CVA or stroke. Unfortunately these stroke-like presentations can also be the result of hypoglycemia. These patients are probably the most important to test blood glucose levels prior to the administration of dextrose. If situation is unclear – consult base physician.

DIAZEPAM (VALIUM)

Pharmacology and actions
Diazepam is a centrally acting agent with properties of an anti-anxiety agent, an anticonvulsant and a skeletal muscle relaxant.

Indications
A. Status epilepticus. In the field, status epilepsy is considered to be any seizure lasting more than 5 minutes, or two consecutive seizures without regaining consciousness.
B. Head trauma. In the patient who is combative and needs sedation to allow for adequate immobilization.
C. Tachydysrhythmias. Prior to cardioversion for the patient who is awake and needs sedation.

Precautions
A. Diazepam can cause respiratory depression or apnea, particularly when given rapidly in children or in patients who have consumed respiratory depressant drugs such as alcohol or barbiturates. Be prepared to assist ventilation if this occurs.
B. Hypotension, and rarely, cardiac arrest may occur with IV use. Monitor patient closely.

Administration – by direct physician order only.
A. Secure the IV line and set out bag-valve-mask prior to administration.
B. Dose – *Adult* – 5–10 mg slow IV push (5 mg/min).

   Pediatric – 2–5 mg slow IV push (0.2 mg/kg).
C. May be administered rectally, if unable to establish IV route, or may be administered IM (with slower onset of effect).

Side effects and special notes
A. In the awake patient, common side effects include drowsiness, dizziness, fatigue and ataxia. Paradoxical excitement or stimulation sometimes occurs.
B. Diazepam should not be mixed with other agents or diluted with IV solutions. Turn off IV flow while administering and give through the end of the IV tubing nearest to the patient.

DIPHENHYDRAMINE (BENADRYL)

Pharmacology and actions
A. An antihistamine which blocks action of histamine released from cells during an allergic reaction.

B. Direct CNS effects which may be stimulant, or more commonly, depressant, depending on individual variation.

C. Anticholinergic, antiparkinsonian effect, which is used to treat acute dystonic reactions to antipsychotic drugs (e.g., Haldol, Thorazine, Compazine, droperidol). These reactions include – oculogyric crisis, acute torticollis, and facial grimacing.

Indications
A. The second-line drug in anaphylaxis and severe allergic reactions (after epinephrine).

B. To counteract acute dystonic reactions to antipsychotic drugs.

Precautions
May have additive effect with alcohol or other depressants.

Administration – by direct physician order only.

A. *Adult* – 50 mg slow IV push or deep IM.

B. *Pediatric* – 2 mg/kg slow IV or deep IM (not to exceed 50 mg total).

Side effects and special notes
A. Benadryl is not the first line drug for allergic reactions, but may be useful for long transports.

B. Benadryl may also be useful for acute dystonic reactions. These reactions can be emotionally and physically trying, but are seldom life-threatening. It may allow transport of a less agitated and anxious patient.

C. Benadryl occasionally is used prophylactically with droperidol to increase sedation, and decrease the risk of dystonic reactions.

DOPAMINE (INTROPIN)

Pharmacology and actions

Dopamine is a chemical precursor of norepinephrine. It occurs naturally in man, and has both alpha and beta receptor stimulating actions, as well as action on specific dopaminergic receptors. At high doses, actions are very similar to those of norepinephrine (Levophed). At lower dose levels, the differential effects allow cardiac stimulation and support of blood pressure without increasing oxygen demand and vasoconstricting vital organs as much as earlier vasopressors. In general, the following actions are seen:

A. 1–2 mcg/kg/min – dilates renal and mesenteric blood vessels (no effect on heart rate or blood pressure).

B. 2–10 mcg/kg/min – beta effects on heart usually increase cardiac output without increasing heart rate or blood pressure.

C. 10–20 mcg/kg/min – alpha peripheral effects causes peripheral vasoconstriction and increased blood pressure.

D. 20–40 mcg/kg/min – alpha effects reverse dilatation of renal and mesenteric vessels with resultant decreased flow.

Indications

A. Hypotension which is hemodynamically significant in the *absence* of hypovolemia (i.e., cardiogenic shock).

B. Septic or neurogenic shock when unresponsive to other measures (secondary use only).

Precautions

A. *Dopamine is contraindicated in hypovolemic shock.* Pressor agents make tissue hypoxia worse in the presence of hypovolemia. Because even some cardiac patients may be hypovolemic from diuretics and poor fluid intake, careful evaluation is necessary. Invasive monitoring is often the only way to differentiate forms of shock in the elderly and treatment with dopamine is, therefore, indicated in the field only in severely unstable patients with evidence of increased venous pressure.

B. Dopamine is best administered by an infusion pump to accurately regulate rate. This is another reason it is hazardous for field use. *Monitor closely.*

C. May induce tachydysrhythmias, in which case, infusion should be decreased or stopped.

D. At low doses, decreased blood pressure may occur due to peripheral vasodilatation. Increasing infusion rate will correct this.

E. Should not be added to sodium bicarbonate or other alkaline solutions since dopamine will be inactivated at higher pH.

Administration – by direct physician order only.
A. Mix – 400 mg (2 ampules) in 250 ml D5W (or use premixed) to produce concentration of 1600 mcg/ml.

B. *Adult* – IV infusion only. Start at 5 mcg/kg/min. Increase by 5 mcg/kg/min every 2–3 minutes to a level of 10–20 mcg/kg/min to achieve desired effect. Microdrip chamber only.

C. *Pediatric* – Not appropriate for prehospital use.

Side effects and special notes
A. Most common side effects include ectopic beats, nausea and vomiting. Angina has also been reported following treatment. Tachycardia and dysrhythmias occur but are less likely than with older pressor agents.

B. Dopamine "whips" the heart and increases oxygen consumption, although to a lesser extent than other catecholamines. It should be reserved for patients with serious symptomatic hypotension NOT caused by hypovolemia.

C. Tissue extravasation at the IV site can cause skin sloughing due to vasoconstriction. Be sure to make emergency department personnel aware if there has been any extravasation so proper treatment can be instituted.

D. Can cause hypertensive crisis.

E. Certain antidepressants potentiate the effects of this drug. Check for medications and contact base if other medications are being used.

TABLE 8-1.   INTRAVENOUS DRIP RATES FOR DOPAMINE

Concentration – 1600 mcg/ml
Drip Rate – microdrips/min

Weight (kg)	Dose (mcg/kg/min)			
	5	10	15	20
50	10	20	30	40 microdrip/min
60	10	25	35	45
70	15	25	40	50
80	15	30	45	60
90	15	35	50	70
100	20	35	55	75
110	20	40	60	85

Drip rates in table do not yield *exact* mcg/kg/min, but are very close and are useful for field application.

DROPERIDOL (INAPSINE)

Pharmacology and actions
Droperidol is one of the butyrophenone series of major tranquilizers. The effects include antianxiety, mild sedation, and neuroleptic reactions. Neuroleptic syndrome consists of suppression of spontaneous movements and complex behavior – while spinal reflexes and unconditioned nociceptive-avoidance behavior remains intact. In man, neuroleptic drugs reduce initiative and interest in the environment, and they reduce displays of emotion or affect. The precise mechanism of action has not been established. Droperidol also has strong antiemetic properties.

Indications
A. The primary field indication is in the management of manifestations of acute psychosis: severe agitation, hyperactivity, combativeness, hostility, negativism, and hallucinations. The antipsychotic drugs are not specific for the diagnostic type of psychosis to be treated, and are effective in a wide range of disorders in which psychotic symptoms and severe agitation are prominent.

B. Secondary field use is for intractable nausea and vomiting with prolonged transport time.

Precautions
A. Administer with caution to patients with history of severe cardiovascular disease – may produce hypotension or angina. Fluids should be available to treat hypotension, which is a common side effect. Epinephrine is not effective in treating this complication, due to the alpha blocking properties of droperidol, and may paradoxically make the hypotension worse. QT prolongation has been reported and at least one report of torsade de pointes.

B. As with other neuroleptic drugs there is a rare occurrence of neuroleptic malignant syndrome (altered level of consciousness, muscle rigidity, and autonomic instability). Notify base hospital immediately with any high fever or tachydysrhythmias.

Administration – by direct physician order only.
A. Two ml ampule – 2.5 mg/ml.

B. *Adult* – If IV has been established 0.05–0.1 mg/kg may be administered IV. Rapid effect (5–10 minutes) should be apparent.

C. If unable to establish IV due to extreme agitation, administer 0.1 mg/kg IM in any convenient large muscle mass. Effect will be more delayed than IV route (15–20 minutes).

D. Dosage for intractable nausea and vomiting should be half the above dose (0.025 – 0.05 mg/kg) IV.

E. *Pediatric* – Not for field use in children.

Side effects and special notes

A. Droperidol, like other major tranquilizers of the phenothiazine class, can produce significant extrapyramidal symptoms within 12–48 hours. Spasm of the muscles of tongue, face, neck, and back are the most common. The symptoms can be mild or severe – with opisthotonos or oculogyric crisis. Benadryl 50 mg IV may decrease the risk of these reactions which are idiosyncratic *not* allergic. The risk of these reactions with droperidol are considerably less than the related drug, haloperidol.

B. Multiple other neurological effects of these (neuroleptic) drugs include parkinsonism, akathisia, tardive dyskinesia, and Neuroleptic malignant syndrome. These complications occur with prolonged treatment regimens, *not* with one-time emergency use of droperidol.

C. Hyperpyrexia and heat stroke may be an uncommon, but abrupt complication.

D. As with all tranquilizing drugs, the effects with other sedatives are additive and there is always the possibility of respiratory depression. Should only be administered when patient will be under close observation with airway adjuncts at hand.

EPINEPHRINE

Pharmacology and actions
A. Catecholamine with alpha (α) and beta (β) effects.

B. In general, the following cardiovascular responses can be expected:

1. Increased heart rate.

2. Increased myocardial contractile force.

3. Increased systemic vascular resistance.

4. Increased arterial blood pressure.

5. Increased myocardial O_2 consumption.

6. Increased automaticity of the heart.

C. Potent bronchodilatation.

D. Pupillary dilatation.

The primary effect of epinephrine in cardiac arrest is peripheral vasoconstriction, which leads to improved coronary and cerebral perfusion pressure. It seems to produce beneficial redistribution of blood from peripheral to central circulation during CPR. It also seems to make ventricular fibrillation more responsive to countershock.

Indications
A. Ventricular fibrillation or pulseless ventricular tachycardia, unresponsive to initial countershocks.

B. Asystole.

C. Pulseless Electrical Activity (PEA).

D. Bradycardia with signs of shock.

E. Systemic allergic reactions or anaphylaxis.

F. Asthma.

Precautions
A. Should not be added directly to bicarbonate infusion, since catecholamines may be partially inactivated by alkaline solution.

B. When used for allergic reactions, increased cardiac work can precipitate angina or MI in susceptible individuals.

C. Due to peripheral vasoconstriction, should be used with caution in patients with poor peripheral circulation.

D. Wheezing in an elderly person is more often due to pulmonary edema (pulmonary embolus is also a possible cause). Epinephrine is not indicated for pulmonary edema.

E. Because epinephrine is a non-selective β drug, it exerts considerable stimulation effect on the heart. In asthma, particularly in older patients with heart disease, this may be detrimental and a more selective bronchodilator should be used if possible.

Administration

Adult

A. Cardiac arrest – 1.0 mg (10 ml of 1:10,000 solution) IV initially, then 1.0 mg IV every 3–5 minutes thereafter, or give first dose 2.5 mg (2.5 ml of *1:1000*) via endotracheal tube. Flush each IV dose with 20 ml fluid bolus.

B. Anaphylactic shock, laryngeal edema – 1 ml of 1:10,000 SLOW IV or epinephrine drip.

C. By direct physician order:

    1. Generalized allergic reaction (with adequate perfusion) – 0.3 mg (0.3 ml of *1:1,000* solution) SQ.

    2. Asthma – 0.3 mg (0.3 ml of *1:1,000* solution) SQ. In patients over 40 years of age, use only for severe respiratory distress.

    3. To enhance adrenergic tone – Epinephrine drip 1 to 4 mg in 250 D5W, to start at 1 mcg/min, titrate to effect.

Pediatric

A. Cardiac arrest – 0.01 mg/kg (0.1 ml/kg of 1:10,0000) IV or 0.1 mg/kg via ET tube (0.1 ml/kg of *1:1000 – ten times the IV dose*). Repeat IV dose every 3–5 minutes during the arrest. Flush each IV dose with 5–10 ml fluid bolus.

B. By direct physician order:

    1. Generalized allergic reaction (with adequate perfusion) – 0.01 mg/kg (0.01 ml/kg of *1:1,000* solution) SQ.

2. Asthma – 0.01 mg/kg (0.01 ml/kg of *1:1,000*) SQ.

3. Bradycardia associated with signs of shock and unresponsive to airway improvement – 0.01 mg/kg (0.1 ml/kg of 1:10,000) IV.

Side effects and special notes

A. Anxiety, tremor, palpitations, and headache are common side effects.

B. *Relatively* contraindicated in patients with hypertension, hyperthyroidism, angina, or cerebrovascular insufficiency.

C. Epinephrine is one prehospital drug that comes in two different strengths. The doses in milligrams are the same, but the volume of solution is different. Errors can be very dangerous (by a factor of 10).

D. Epinephrine is extremely potent when given IV. It is easy to become cavalier since we commonly treat the cardiac arrest patient with "mega-dose" epinephrine. The effects on a *live* person with an intact cardiovascular system (even compromised by anaphylaxis) are significantly different. Epinephrine should be given IV in a *live* adult patient only in 1 ml (1:10,000) increments (0.1 mg) to prevent excess hypertension and dysrhythmias.

E. The use of high doses of epinephrine for the patient in cardiac arrest has had some recent support. So far, the data indicates it is able to produce electrical rhythms far more effectively than actually saving lives. The AHA has left it labeled as "not specifically recommended; acceptable, possibly helpful". The exact drug dosage is appropriate for direct physician order.

F. Basic prehospital care personnel may assist with administration of the patient's Epi-pen or anaphylaxis kit after direction from base physician.

FUROSEMIDE (LASIX)

Pharmacology and actions
Furosemide is a potent diuretic with a rapid onset of action and short duration of effect. It acts primarily by inhibiting sodium reabsorption throughout the kidney. Increase in potassium excretion occurs along with the sodium excretion. As an IV bolus, it causes immediate (3–4 minutes) increase in venous capacitance. This decreases venous back-up and probably accounts for an immediate effect in pulmonary edema. Peak effect is $^1/_2$–1 hour after IV administration; duration about 2 hours. Duration 6–8 hours if given orally, with a peak in 1–2 hours. Tolerance develops and larger doses may be needed in patients with renal failure or those chronically taking furosemide.

Indications
A. Acute pulmonary edema – to decrease extracellular volume and reduce venous pressure in the lungs in cardiac failure.
B. Massive head trauma – used in some regions to treat traumatic cerebral edema and lower intracranial pressure.

Precautions
A. Do not use in presence of hypotension (systolic BP < 90) or other signs of hypovolemia. Can lead to profound diuresis with resultant shock and electrolyte depletion.
B. Have urinal available. Effect may be seen within 10–15 minutes.
C. Foley catheter insertion should be performed during long transports (over 30 minutes) or before transferring a head-injured patient receiving diuretics, in order to prevent bladder injury or incontinence.

Administration – by direct physician order only.
A. *Adult dose* – 20–40 mg slowly IV (over 2 minutes). 1 ampule = 2 ml = 20 mg.
B. *Pediatric dose* – 1 mg/kg.

Side effects and special notes
A. Because of potency and need for close monitoring, should only be used in the field in seriously ill patients who require immediate intervention.

B. Dose of furosemide may need to be increased in patients chronically taking furosemide. Check with base if you think a larger dose may be indicated.

C. May cause acute and profound diarrhea.

D. Hypokalemia, hyponatremia, and hypovolemia are the main toxic effects. The hypokalemia is of particular concern in digitalized patients, and especially in digitalis-toxic patients.

GLUCAGON

Pharmacology and actions

Glucagon is a hormone which causes glucose mobilization in the body. It works opposite to insulin, which causes glucose storage, and it is normally secreted in the pancreas. Glucagon is released at times of insult or injury when glucose is needed. It stimulates the synthesis of cyclic AMP and its metabolic effects are similar to epinephrine. In the hypoglycemic patient, return to consciousness will be about 20 minutes after IM dose.

Indications

A. Hypoglycemia or insulin shock in patients who are unconscious (unable to take oral solutions) and in whom venous access cannot be obtained.

B. Hypoglycemia in combative, uncontrollable patient in whom IV dextrose cannot be administered and transport time is over 20 minutes.

C. To increase myocardial contractility in patients with critically symptomatic Beta blocker or calcium channel blocker overdose.

Precautions

A. Patients with no liver glycogen stores (due to alcoholism, malnutrition) may not be able to mobilize any glucose in response to glucagon and the treatment will be ineffective.

B. Hyperglycemic effect of glucagon is of short duration (1–2 hour) so the patient must be transported and fed to replenish glucose stores and prevent recurrence of the hypoglycemia.

Administration – by direct physician order only.

A. *Adults* – Hypoglycemia – 1.0 mg IM or SQ.

        Beta blocker overdose – 2–4 mg IV (MUST BE DILUTED WITH D5W FOR THIS PURPOSE, NOT THE DILUENT PROVIDED WHICH CONTAINS PHENOL.)

B. *Children* under 12 years – 0.5 mg IM or SQ.

Side effects and special notes

A. Nausea and vomiting may occur.

B. IV glucose or dextrose is the treatment of choice for insulin shock. Use of glucagon is restricted to patients as described above in whom IV access is impossible. In these rare situations, it can be very useful.

IPECAC

Pharmacology and actions
Ipecac alkaloids act both locally on the gastric mucosa and centrally on the chemoreceptor trigger zone to induce vomiting. Usually effective within 20–30 minutes.

Indications
To induce vomiting in patients who have ingested poisons or drugs. Should be used only in regions where there is Poison Control Center (PCC) or local physician endorsement.

Precautions
A. Contraindications:

1. Patients who are unconscious or with diminishing level of consciousness.

2. Patients who are actively seizing.

3. Patients who have ingested acids, alkalis, silver nitrate, iodides, or strychnine.

B. Ipecac syrup should not be confused with Ipecac *fluid extract*. The latter is very concentrated and has caused death when ingested.

Administration – by direct physician (or PCC) order.

A. *Adult* – 30 ml orally.

B. *Pediatric* (over one year) – 15 ml orally.

Side effects and special notes
A. The emetic action is improved if fluids are given orally just before or after the ipecac (2–3 glasses of water in adults).

B. Emetic action may be enhanced by walking.

C. The gag reflex may be an unreliable indicator of whether or not someone will be able to protect the airway in the event of emesis. Additionally, testing for a gag reflex in a patient with depressed level of consciousness may actually cause vomiting and subsequent aspiration. *Use caution.*

D. Always stand by with suction. Patient should be supported on their side (lateral decubitus position). Monitor carefully for decreasing level of consciousness and vomiting.

IV SOLUTIONS

Pharmacology and actions
Two types of solutions are available for use in the field.

A. Volume expanders (Ringer's lactate or normal saline)

   These contain sodium as the major cation and expand the extracellular fluid space. RL is the same tonicity (concentration of electrolytes) as body fluids. NS is actually slightly hypertonic.

B. Water solution (D5W)

   This diffuses through three times the body space of NS and RL. It is therefore, inefficient as a volume expander. Dextrose contained in the solution makes it isotonic to body cells and prevents solution from damaging cells. The dextrose is rapidly metabolized and produces little energy for the body to use (200 cal/L). The net effect is addition of water to the patient.

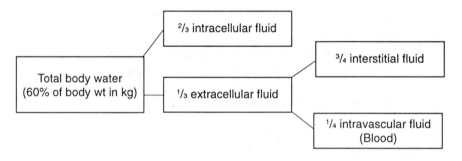

When replacing fluids:

Blood – stays in intravascular space.

Volume expander (RL or NS) – diffuses through extracellular volume ($^1/_4$ stays intravascular).

Water (D5W) – diffuses through total body water ($^1/_{12}$ stays intravascular).

Indications
A. Volume expanders – to expand intravascular volume in the presence of hemorrhagic shock, volume depletion (dehydration, burns, severe vomiting), or shock caused by increased vascular space (neurogenic shock).

B. Water solutions – to obtain intravenous access to a patient.

    1. To treat with IV medications.

    2. To assure later access for treatment in patients with potentially unstable conditions.

Precautions

A. In hemorrhagic shock, volume expansion with *blood* is the treatment of choice. Crystalloid solutions (RL or NS) will temporarily expand intravascular volume and "buy time", but do not increase oxygen-carrying capacity, and are insufficient in severe shock. Because of this, rapid transport is still necessary to treat severely hypovolemic patients who need blood and possibly surgical intervention to stop ongoing bleeding.

B. Volume overload is a constant danger, particularly in cardiac patients. Keep a close eye on your IV rate during transport. Mysterious excess fluid boluses are all too common. Consider saline lock if fluid is not required.

Administration

A. Through peripheral vein by needle or cannula.

B. TKO = 20–40 microdrips/min = 5–10 drops/min. Rate to be used for all D5W IVs and stable patients with volume expanders.

C. For administration of fluid bolus – 20 ml/kg volume expander through large bore cannula, as rapidly as possible.

D. 1 ml/min = 60 microdrops/min = 15 regular drops/min.

E. Needle or cannula size: 25 gauge = smallest
                                14 gauge = largest

For administration of volume expanders (RL or NS) – largest diameter possible (14 gauge preferred).

For administration of water solutions – size not as important; aim for security and accuracy. Larger bore can occasionally be useful.

Side effects and special notes

A. TKO rate should always be used for water solutions *and* for volume expanders in a stable patient. Without excess fluids, you will know that your patient is stable and not being "helped" by fluids. Give wide open bolus as above if fluids are needed.

B. In trauma patients, 14 g cannulas should be used most frequently. Flow rate through a 14 g cannula is twice the rate through an 18 g cannula, and volume administration in trauma patients can be accomplished more rapidly. The larger cannula is more painful to insert, but with practice can be placed reliably. If the patient has poor veins, a smaller bore is better than no IV at all in most instances.

C. IVs in an unstable trauma patient should be placed en route, and may be left to the hospital setting for short transports. Do not delay transport for IV attempts.

D. Two attempts are the limit per person. If you are unable to start in two attempts, another qualified attendant may try, or leave the IVs for the hospital. Some patients are very difficult and some days are more difficult too!

E. IV fluid bolus for the trauma patient in shock is increasingly controversial. Recent data question the wisdom of pouring fluids into a patient who has ongoing blood loss internally. Patients at risk for internal hemorrhage should have two large bore lines. By system consensus volume expander may be kept at TKO rate until the patient is in the hospital (ED or OR) where internal bleeding can be controlled. After bleeding is controlled, those lines may prove invaluable for infusing fluids and blood.

LIDOCAINE (XYLOCAINE)

Pharmacology and actions

A. Depresses automaticity of Purkinje fibers; therefore, raises stimulation threshold in the ventricular muscle fibers (makes ventricles less likely to fibrillate).

B. Little antidysrhythmic effect on atrial muscle at subtoxic levels.

C. May suppress cough reflex at therapeutic levels. This will result in decreased intracerebral pressure response to intubation.

D. CNS stimulation: tremor, restlessness and clonic convulsions, followed by depression and respiratory failure at higher doses.

E. Cardiovascular effects: decreased conduction rate and force of contraction, mainly at toxic levels.

F. The effect of a single bolus on the heart disappears in 10–20 minutes due to redistribution in the body. Metabolic half-life is about 2 hours; therefore, toxicity develops with repeated doses.

Indications

A. Significant PVCs in suspected myocardial infarction or contusion when:

   1. PVCs more than 6/minute.

   2. Close coupled PVCs (R on T).

   3. Multifocal PVCs.

   4. Runs of 2 or more PVCs in a row.

B. Ventricular tachycardia or wide-complex tachycardia with pulses.

C. Recurrent or refractory ventricular fibrillation.

D. Following successful defibrillation in patients prone to recurrent ventricular fibrillation.

E. Prior to intubation in patients suspected of having increased intracranial pressure.

F. Prior to intubation in patients at risk for vagal mediated cardiac dysrhythmias.

Precautions

A. Use with extreme caution in presence of advanced A-V block unless artificial pacemaker is in place.

B. Atrial fibrillation or flutter, quinidine-like effect may cause alarming ventricular acceleration.

C. Lidocaine is not recommended for treatment of supraventricular rhythms.

D. Diazepam should be available to treat convulsions if they occur.

E. Do not treat ventricular escape beats with lidocaine. In severe block, these may be providing patient perfusion.

F. Do not delay intubation efforts to start an IV or administer medication when the primary need is AIRWAY.

Administration
Intermittent bolus method – for cardiac arrest.
A. *Adult* – 1.5 mg/kg IV bolus.

   Pediatric – 1 mg/kg IV bolus.

B. Second bolus of 0.5 mg/kg IV after 5–10 minutes for persistent VF.

C. Third bolus of 0.5 mg/kg given after another 5–10 min during long transports with persistent VF. Max 3 mg/kg by bolus only.

Bolus and drip method –to treat *significant* PVCs in patient with good circulation.
A. 1 mg/kg slow IV bolus, **adult and pediatric.**

B. 2nd bolus of 0.5 mg/kg IV is given 5–10 minutes after 1st bolus in addition to drip. Max 3 mg/kg by repeat bolus.

C. IV drip – Mix 1 gm lidocaine in 250 ml D5W for a concentration of 4 mg/ml (or use premixed drip solution, 2 gm lidocaine in 250 ml for concentration of 8 mg/ml). Run 2–4 mg/min (20–40 mcg/kg/min) or 30–60 microdrops/min. Must be started soon after first bolus or blood levels will rapidly disappear.

Single bolus dosing – for intubation.
   Single IV dose (1.5 mg/kg) if time available in comatose patient who needs intubation. Administer just 60 seconds before intubation.

Note – Bolus (to 3 mg/kg) may be administered through endotracheal tube.

Side effects

A. CNS disturbances – sleepiness, dizziness, disorientation, confusion, muscular twitching, focal or grand mal seizures.

B. Hypotension – increased A-V block and decreased myocardial contractility at toxic levels only.

C. Rare instances of sudden cardiovascular collapse and death.

D. Toxicity is increased in elderly patients and those with liver impairment.

Special notes

A. Lidocaine is metabolized in the liver and elderly patients and patients with hepatic disease, shock or congestive heart failure will not break down the drug rapidly. Administer 1.0 mg/kg and reduce the drip by one-half. Second bolus usually not indicated.

B. A bolus of lidocaine will establish a given level of drug in the blood. The drip maintains this level by replacing metabolized drug. It should, therefore, be started rapidly. Without a bolus, a drip has no effect for 30–60 minutes. The second bolus is given to prevent an observed dip in blood level which occurs 20 minutes after initial bolus and drip.

C. Lidocaine is another drug which comes in several different solutions for prehospital use.

Prefilled syringes – 50–100 mg in 5–10 ml for bolus administration (1% solution).

Vials – 500–1000 mg in 5–10 ml solution for IV drips (10% solution).

Premixed drip solution – 2 gm in 250 ml D5W for concentration of 8 mg/ml.

D. The desire to treat all PVCs is a disease called the "lidocaine itch". It is commonly found in field and hospital personnel. PVCs should be treated only when significant and premature ventricular beats are encountered in the setting of acute angina or MI. PVCs generated by hypoxia will not respond to lidocaine and the wrong life-threat will be treated.

E. Prophylactic lidocaine in the patient with cardiac type chest pain is no longer recommended. The patient with chest pain who is also having frequent or multifocal PVCs, however, should have lidocaine administered to treat PVCs. This is not the same as prophylactic use (giving the drug before it is needed to prevent it being needed). Do not hesitate to treat dangerous PVCs in the patient with suspected cardiac chest pain.

MAGNESIUM SULFATE

Pharmacology and actions

Magnesium is a cofactor for many enzymatic reactions. It is essential for the function of the sodium-potassium ATPase pump. Magnesium prevents or controls convulsions by blocking neuromuscular transmissions. Magnesium has a depressant effect on the CNS. It acts as a physiological calcium channel blocker and may also produce heart block. Magnesium may reduce the incidence of post infarction ventricular dysrhythmias.

Indications

A. Pregnant patients (usually greater than 20 weeks) with severe preeclampsia.

   1. Blood pressure greater than 180 systolic or 120 diastolic.

   2. Altered mental status.

   3. Generalized or severe localized edema.

   4. Headache and/or visual disturbance.

B. Pregnant patients (usually greater than 20 weeks) with eclampsia – any of the above signs *and* seizures.

C. May be useful in allowing conversion of ventricular tachycardia or fibrillation unresponsive to defibrillation, epinephrine, lidocaine or bretylium.

D. Treatment of choice for torsades de pointes.

E. May be useful for the treatment of asthma which is severe and not responding promptly to albuterol.

Precautions

A. May occasionally lead to A-V blocks or respiratory arrest. Calcium chloride may reverse respiratory and cardiac effects. Calcium should be readily available before administration of magnesium sulfate.

B. Not indicated in patients with heart block or significant cardiac disease. (Use caution if patient is taking digitalis.)

Administration – by direct physician order only.

Administer 1–2 gm in 50 ml D5W to run in over 15–20 minutes.

Side effects and special notes

A. Principle complication is respiratory depression. Be prepared. Never administer as a bolus.

B. May need to decrease dosage if patient is using other depressant drugs (e.g., barbiturates, narcotics, hypnotics). Effects may be additive and increase the risk of respiratory depression.

MORPHINE SULFATE (MS)

Pharmacology and actions
A. Analgesia.

B. Pupil constriction.

C. Respiration – decreased rate and tidal volume.

D. Peripheral vasodilatation.

E. Cardiac effect (reflex due to vasodilatation):

    1. Decreased myocardial oxygen consumption.

    2. Decreased left ventricular end-diastolic pressure.

    3. Decreased cardiac work.

    4. May decrease incidence of dysrhythmias.

F. Effect – maximum within 7 minutes IV.

Indications
A. Presumed cardiac chest pain – usually severe, typically crushing or pressing substernal, often a sweaty patient who looks sick.

B. Isolated extremity fractures when severe pain is present. To be given only with no evidence of head, chest or abdominal injuries.

C. Back and neck injuries when sedation/pain relief are necessary to prevent a patient from moving around and potentially injuring himself.

D. Acute pulmonary edema.

Precautions
A. Hypotension is a relative contraindication to use of morphine. *Remember that some people will be hypotensive in response to pain itself.* Smaller doses are less likely to cause or aggravate hypotension.

B. Head injuries or abdominal injuries are also relative contraindications to morphine use, since the analgesic effect removes the clinical signs that need to be watched. With a combative head injured patient, however, it may be far safer than physical violence. Discuss with base physician.

C. Do not use in person with respiratory difficulties (except pulmonary edema) because their respiratory drive may become depressed.

D. Do not use in the presence of major blood loss. The body's compensatory mechanisms will be suppressed by the use of morphine and the hypotensive effect will become very prominent.

E. May cause vomiting. Administer slowly.

Administration – by direct physician order only.
A. IV only (unless you cannot start an IV and are specifically directed to administer IM).

B. *Adult* – 2–4 mg IV initially, repeat every 5 minutes if needed. Do not exceed 0.2 mg/kg. The goal is decreased anxiety and patient comfort. The patient need not be completely pain-free.

C. *Pediatric* – 0.1 mg/kg slowly IV.

Side effects and special notes
A. The major side effects and complications from morphine result from vasodilatation. This causes no problems if the patient is supine and not volume depleted. It may cause problems if the patient is upright, hypovolemic, or has decreased cardiac output (after MI).

B. Allergic reactions are rare, but ask! If patient reports allergy to other narcotics – ask for the reaction. Codeine notoriously causes nausea, vomiting, or GI distress. These are not *allergic* reactions and should have no effect on your use of morphine. The patient who reports allergies to many narcotics and reports swelling of the airway, shock, or other significant responses, however, *should not* receive morphine.

C. Be prepared to ventilate if the patient stops breathing. Naloxone can be used to reverse medication effects, but it leaves no good alternative for pain relief. Respiratory support may be a better alternative.

NALOXONE (NARCAN)

Pharmacology and actions
Naloxone is a narcotic antagonist which competitively binds to narcotic sites but which exhibits almost no pharmacologic activity of its own. Duration of action is 1–4 hours.

Indications
A. Reversal of narcotic effects, particularly respiratory depression due to narcotic drugs either ingested, injected or administered in the course of treatment. Narcotic drugs include morphine, Demerol, heroin, Dilaudid, Percodan, codeine, Lomotil, propoxyphene (Darvon), or pentazocine (Talwin).

B. Diagnostically in coma of unknown etiology to detect or reverse narcotic cardiorespiratory depression if present.

C. Seizure of unknown etiology to reverse possible narcotic overdose (particularly propoxyphene).

D. May reverse vasodepressant and cardiac depressant substances present in septic or hypovolemic shock.

Precautions
A. In patients who are addicted to narcotics, frank and occasionally violent withdrawal symptoms may be precipitated. Titrate the dose (0.2 ml at a time) to reverse cardiac and respiratory depression but keep the patient groggy. Be prepared to restrain the patient.

B. Titration may also assist the patient who is taking narcotics for pain (patients with known cancer). Very small amounts over time can reverse the respiratory depression, but still leave the patient with some pain control.

C. May need large doses (8–12 mg) to reverse propoxyphene (Darvon) overdose.

Administration
A. Supplied in various concentrations. Stock and use only one, if possible, to avoid confusion or drug errors.

    1 ml ampule = 0.4 mg.
    2 ml ampule = 2.0 mg.
    10 ml vial = 4.0 mg.

B. *Adult* – 2 mg IV, repeat as needed.
   Pediatric – 0.04 mg/kg IV.

C. If no response is observed, this dose may be repeated after 5 minutes if narcotic overdose is strongly suspected.

Side effects and special notes

A. This drug is remarkably safe and free from side effects. Do not hesitate to use it if indicated.

B. The duration of some narcotics is longer than naloxone. The patient must be monitored closely since repeated doses of naloxone may be necessary. Patients who have received this drug *must be transported* to the hospital since coma may recur as naloxone wears off.

C. With an endotracheal tube in place and assisted ventilation, narcotic overdose patients may be safely managed without naloxone. Think twice before totally reversing coma. Airway control may be lost, or worse, the patient may refuse transport.

NITROGLYCERIN

Pharmacology and actions

A. Cardiovascular effects include:

1. Reduced venous tone, causing blood-pooling in peripheral veins and decreasing venous return to the heart.

2. Decreased peripheral resistance.

3. Dilatation of coronary arteries (if not already at maximum) and relief of coronary artery spasm.

B. Generalized smooth muscle relaxation (including esophagus).

Indications

A. Angina.

B. Chest, arm, or neck pain thought caused by coronary ischemia.

C. Control of hypertension in angina or acute MI.

D. Pulmonary edema – to increase venous pooling, lowering cardiac preload and afterload.

Precautions

A. Generalized vasodilatation may cause profound hypotension and reflex tachycardia.

B. NTG loses potency easily. It should be stored in dark glass container with tight lid and not exposed to heat.

C. Use with caution in hypotensive patients.

Administration

A. *Adult* – 0.4 mg (1/150) tablet sublingually. May repeat every 5 minutes as needed for effect.

B. Nitroglycerin spray (0.4 mg) may be used as alternative.

C. *Pediatric* – Not indicated for use in children.

Side effects and special notes

A. Common side effects include throbbing headache, flushing, dizziness and burning under the tongue. These side effects may be used to check potency of medication.

B. Less common – orthostatic hypotension, sometimes marked. Be prepared to lay patient flat and elevate legs if blood pressure drops.

C. Note: Therapeutic effect is enhanced but adverse effects are increased when patient is upright.

D. Because nitroglycerin causes generalized smooth muscle relaxation, it may be effective in relieving chest pain caused by esophageal spasm.

E. May be effective even in patients using paste, discs, or oral long-acting nitrate preparations.

F. Repeated nitroglycerin administration, even when patient is pain-free, may be used to control blood pressure and decrease cardiac work.

G. Basic prehospital care personnel may assist with administration of the patient's nitroglycerin after direction from base physician.

OXYGEN

Pharmacology and actions

Oxygen added to the inspired air raises the amount of oxygen in the blood, and therefore, the amount delivered to the tissues. Tissue hypoxia causes cell damage and death. Breathing in most persons is regulated by small changes in acid/base balance and CO_2 levels. It takes relatively large drops in blood O_2 concentration to stimulate respiration.

Indications

A. Respiratory distress or suspected hypoxemia from any cause.

B. Chest pain in which myocardial ischemia or infarction is suspected.

C. Shock (decreased oxygenation of tissues) from any cause.

D. Major trauma.

E. Carbon monoxide poisoning.

F. Any inhalation or noxious gas exposure.

G. High altitude illness.

Precautions

A. If the patient is not breathing adequately on his own, the treatment should be ventilation, not just O_2. A nasal cannula without a breath is a waste of O_2 (and patients)!

B. A *small* percentage of patients with chronic lung disease breathe because they are hypoxic. Administration of O_2 may shut off their respiratory drive. *Do not withhold oxygen because of this possibility. Be prepared to assist ventilation if needed.* Initial O_2 flow should be 2 L/min or 1 L/min greater than home O_2 in these patients.

C. If pulse oximetry is available, titrate oxygen saturation (SaO_2) to 90% or greater. Be aware, however, that in some cases, the reading will be meaningless (CO poisoning) and oxygen flow should be at a maximum (10–15 L/min). In patients with COPD, pulse oximetry may not reach 90% even with high flow, non-rebreather mask. Titrate to patient comfort or pulse oximetry greater than 80% if possible.

Administration

Dosage: Indications:

Low flow (1–2 L/min)   Patients with chronic lung disease.

Moderate flow (4–6 L/min)   Minimal respiratory difficulty. Trauma.
                                 Abdominal pain.

High flow (10–15 L/min)   Severe breathing difficulty (medical or
                                 traumatic.) Carbon monoxide poisoning.
                                 Chest pain. Shock. Smoke inhalation.

Side effects and special notes

A. Nonhumidified O_2 is drying and irritating to mucous membranes.

B. Restlessness may be an important sign of hypoxia. Do not let a combative, head-injured patient deter you from application of O_2.

C. On the other hand, some persons become more agitated when a nasal cannula is applied, particularly when it is not needed. Acquiesce to the patient if it is reasonable. Consider alternatives. Nasal cannulas can be applied to the mouth just as easily and may be better tolerated.

D. Oxygen supports combustion but is not flammable.

E. Oxygen toxicity (overdose) is not a hazard from acute administration. However, many patients with respiratory distress will feel quite comfortable with an increase in their inspired O_2 from 21% to 24%. Excessive oxygen is noisy, drying, and empties the tanks rapidly.

F. Nasal prongs work equally well on nose and mouth breathers.

G. The field and hospital treatment for CO poisoning is *100%* oxygen. This is best obtained by a mask with a good fit and a reservoir bag and a high O_2 flow rate. Do not stop O_2 administration after the patient becomes awake and oriented. Considerable levels of CO may still be present in the blood (and cells). If ventilatory assistance is needed, use the method allowing the highest O_2 concentration possible.

H. Children frequently will be frightened by a mask. Nasal prongs may be better tolerated – or let Mom hold the oxygen tubing near the child's face.

TABLE 8-2. OXYGEN CONCENTRATIONS BY VARIOUS METHODS OF ADMINISTRATION

Method	Flow Rate	O_2 in Inspired Air (approximate)
Room air		21%
Nasal cannula (prongs)	1 L/min	24%
	2 L/min	28%
	8 L/min	40%
Face mask	10 L/min	50–60%
Mask with reservoir	10 L/min	90%
Mouth-to-mask	10 L/min	50%
	15 L/min	80%
	30 L/min	100%
Bag-valve-mask	room air	21%
	12 L/min	40%
BVM with reservoir	10–15 L/min	90%
O_2-powered Breathing device	Hand-regulated	100%

OXYTOCIN (PITOCIN)

Pharmacology and actions

A. Hormone which increases electrical and contractile activity in uterine smooth muscle. Oxytocin can initiate or enhance rhythmic contractions at any time during pregnancy, but the uterus is most sensitive at term.

B. Exhibits rapid onset (minutes), very short half-life, rapid inactivation and excretion.

Indications

A. Control of post-partum hemorrhage.

B. Labor augmentation (in-hospital only).

Precautions

A. Prior to administration, the presence of a second fetus must be considered. Administration with fetus in uterus can cause rupture of uterus or death of fetus.

B. Administration should follow delivery of placenta whenever possible.

Administration – by direct physician order only

A. Injectable oxytocin contains 10 USP units (20 mg) per ml.

B. Intravenous dose – 10–20 USP units in 500 ml volume expander (NS or RL). Flow rate of 10–15 drops/min titrated to severity of hemorrhage and uterine response.

C. Intramuscular dose – 10 USP units (1 ml) only if unable to start IV.

Side effects and special notes

A. In large amounts, oxytocin exhibits a transient but marked vasodilating effect and reflex tachycardia.

B. Cramping may become severe and painful. Administration requires close monitoring of patient during transport.

C. Cardiac dysrhythmias may be precipitated or aggravated by oxytocin.

PHENYLEPHRINE (NEO-SYNEPHRINE)

Pharmacology and actions
Phenylephrine nasal spray exhibits primarily alpha-adrenergic stimulation. This can produce moderate to marked vasoconstriction and nasal decongestion. Other alpha effects such as mydriasis and pressor effects may be apparent even with topical use to mucous membranes.

Indications
A. Primarily used prior to nasotracheal intubation to decrease nasal bleeding from intubation trauma.

B. May relieve ear block and pressure pain with altitude changes by decreasing congestion around eustachian ostia.

Precautions
A. Use with caution, or do not use electively, in patient with known hypertension, hyperthyroidism, diabetes mellitus, or cardiovascular disease.

B. The very young or very old patient will be more likely to have idiosyncratic reactions.

Administration
Nasal spray (1%) – 2 drops in each nostril for *adults*. 1 drop in each nostril for *children or elderly*.

Side effects and special notes
A. When used to relieve otitic barotrauma, the best results are from pretreatment before descending in altitude. If descending and patient experiences pain - stay level or ascend to comfort level. Administer spray and wait 5–10 minutes if time is not critical. Descend when patient reports comfort and/or ability to "pop" ears.

B. When used as pretreatment for nasotracheal intubation, the precautions should not cause undue concern. The patient must need airway assistance but not be in extremis. Critical patients should not have care delayed by administration of nasal spray.

RACEMIC EPINEPHRINE (VAPONEFRIN)

Pharmacology and actions

Racemic epinephrine is an epinephrine preparation with a combination of "L" and "D" isomers of epinephrine for use by *inhalation only*. Effects are those of epinephrine. Inhalation causes local effects on the upper airway as well as systemic effects from absorption. Vasoconstriction may reduce swelling in the upper airway and β effects on bronchial smooth muscle may relieve bronchospasm.

Indications

A. Airway obstruction due to croup.

B. Asthma in pediatric patients.

C. Anaphylaxis in pediatric patients without IV access.

Precautions

A. Mask and noise may be frightening to small children. Agitation will aggravate symptoms of respiratory obstruction. Try to enlist the support of parents and child.

B. Try to differentiate croup from epiglottitis by history. Do not use a tongue blade to examine the back of the throat. The diagnosis is frequently difficult in the field, but a critical patient deserves a trial of racemic epinephrine *during* transport. Although used as specific therapy for croup, it may also buy some time in patients with epiglottitis.

C. In the less-than-critical patient, saline alone via nebulizer may bring symptomatic relief from croup.

D. Racemic epinephrine is heat and light sensitive. It should be stored in a dark cool place. Discoloration is an indication to discard medication.

Administration – by direct physician order only

A. *Over 2 years* – 0.5 ml racemic epinephrine + 2 ml saline, via nebulizer driven by O_2 (6–8 L/min) to create fine mist.

B. *2 years or less* – 0.3 ml racemic epinephrine + 2 ml saline, via nebulizer driven by O_2 (6–8 L/min) to create fine mist.

Side effects and special notes

A. Tachycardia and agitation are the most common side effects. Other side effects of parenteral epinephrine may also be seen. (Since these are also the hallmarks of hypoxia, watch the patient very closely!)

B. Nebulizer treatment may cause blanching of the skin of the mask area due to local epinephrine absorption. Reassure parents.

C. Clinical improvement in croup can be dramatic after administration of racemic epinephrine and presentation in the ED may be markedly altered. Rebound worsening of airway has been described. However, recent studies cast doubt on this phenomenon. Some physicians still feel the need to admit any child treated with racemic epinephrine. A decision to use this medication should, therefore, be made by the regional physicians involved in pediatric care. *Field administration should be limited to critical patients* and should be administered during transport so as to avoid unnecessary delays.

D. If respiratory arrest occurs, it is usually due to patient fatigue or laryngeal spasm. Complete obstruction is not usually present. Ventilate the patient, administer O_2 and transport rapidly. If you can ventilate and oxygenate the patient adequately with pocket mask, or BVM, intubation is best left to a specialist in a controlled setting.

E. Recent studies indicate regular epinephrine (L-epinephrine) may be as effective as racemic epinephrine. If racemic epinephrine is not available, use one to two ml of 1:1,000 epinephrine in a nebulizer, and administer as above.

SODIUM BICARBONATE

Pharmacology and actions
Acids are increased when body tissues become hypoxic due to cardiac or respiratory arrest. While respiratory acidosis and mild metabolic acidosis do not require bicarbonate, marked metabolic acidosis may depress cardiac contractility, depress the cardiac response to catecholamines, and may lower the threshold to fibrillation. Sodium bicarbonate is an alkalotic solution which should neutralize acids found in the blood, although the effectiveness of this in improving the outcome of a critical patient has not been clearly demonstrated.

Indications
A. To correct the acidosis found during cardiac arrest and make the heart more receptive to conversion from ventricular fibrillation, asystole, or electromechanical dissociation by normalizing the pH.

B. To reverse the acidosis found in near-drowning victims.

C. To treat the hypotension or dysrhythmias which may occur as complications of tricyclic antidepressant overdoses.

Precautions
A. Addition of too much $NaHCO_3$ may result in alkalosis (pH of blood higher than normal). This is very difficult to reverse and can cause as many problems in resuscitation as acidosis.

B. Should not be given in mixture with catecholamines or calcium.

C. May increase *cerebral* acidosis, especially in diabetics who are ketotic.

Administration
A. Solutions: *Adult* – 8.4% = 1.0 mEq/ml
   Pediatric – 4.2% = 0.5 mEq/ml
   (Either prepackaged or adult solution diluted 1:1 with sterile water.)

B. For cardiac arrest:

   1. *Adult* – 1 mEq/kg (1 ml/kg). Consider 10 minutes after arrest, then consider 0.5 mEq/kg (0.5 ml/kg) every 10 minutes thereafter until blood gases are available.

2. *Pediatric* – 1 mEq/kg (2 ml/kg). Consider 10 minutes after arrest then consider 0.5 mEq/kg (1 ml/kg) every 20 minutes thereafter.

C. For drowning – 0.5 mEq/kg IV, single dose.

D. For tricyclic OD with hypotension or prolonged QRS (> 0.10 second) – 1.0 mEq/kg IV, repeat if needed in 10–15 minutes.

Side effects and special notes

A. Each ampule of bicarbonate contains 44 to 50 mEq of sodium. In persons with cardiac disease, this sodium will increase intravascular volume and may increase work load on the heart.

B. Hyperosmolarity of the blood can occur because the $NaHCO_3$ is concentrated. This results in cerebral impairment.

C. These dosages are a very rough guide. Blood gases should be obtained as soon as possible to direct further therapy.

D. In the presence of a respiratory arrest without cardiac arrest, the treatment of choice is *ventilation* to correct the respiratory acidosis. No $NaHCO_3$ should be given unless prolonged cardiac arrest has also occurred.

E. Acidosis from medical causes (diabetes, kidney failure) develops gradually. Field treatment is rarely indicated because overtreatment with sodium bicarbonate is dangerous and rapid deterioration is unlikely to develop.

F. In children 10 kg or less, half-strength solution is used to avoid the high concentration of the 8.4% solution. Give *slowly* also, to prevent rapid fluid shifts and intracranial pressure changes in infants.

G. Hyperventilation corrects respiratory acidosis by removing CO_2, which is freely diffusable across cellular and organ membranes. There is little data indicating that therapy with buffers (including bicarbonate) improves outcome. Therefore, adequate attention to airway and ventilation for the first 5–10 minutes of any arrest will allow for maximum respiratory compensation of acidosis. Consider bicarbonate administration after approximately 10 minutes of CPR, but other modalities (such as defibrillation, intubation, ventilation, and more than one trial of epinephrine) should be accomplished first.

H. The initial acidosis in the patient who is in cardiac arrest is primarily respiratory. It is usually a mild acidosis that is not deleterious to resuscitation. Since use of sodium bicarbonate has never been shown to improve outcome, it is currently a Class III (not indicated, may be harmful) for hypoxic lactic acidosis. It is considered Class IIb (acceptable, possibly helpful) for continued long arrest interval if intubated or upon return of spontaneous circulation after long arrest interval. It is Class IIa (acceptable, probably helpful) for tricyclic antidepressant overdose or to alkalize the urine in drug overdoses. It is only considered Class I (definitely helpful) for a patient with known hyperkalemia, which will only occur in the prehospital arena when transporting patients from a renal dialysis unit to a near-by hospital.

VERAPAMIL

Pharmacology and action

Verapamil is a derivative of papaverine. It acts as a slow calcium channel blocker with the following clinical effects:

A. Slows conduction and prolongs refractoriness in AV node.

B. Slows ventricular response to atrial flutter and fibrillation.

C. Vasodilator effect on vascular smooth muscle, including coronary arteries.

D. Negative inotrope, which decreases myocardial oxygen consumption.

Indications

A. Treatment of paroxysmal supraventricular tachycardia (PSVT) in unstable patient who does not require cardioversion.

B. May be useful to slow the ventricular response to atrial flutter or fibrillation in symptomatic patients.

Precautions

A. Vagal maneuvers and adenosine are safer and should be attempted before verapamil is considered.

B. Not for use in patients who are hemodynamically unstable with severe hypotension or congestive heart failure. Patients who appear critical with rapid, narrow complex tachydysrhythmias should be CARDIOVERTED IMMEDIATELY.

C. Verapamil should be used with caution or avoided in patients who are taking beta-adrenergic blocking agents.

D. Contraindicated in patients with sick sinus syndrome or AV block in the absence of a functional artificial pacemaker.

E. Contraindicated for atrial flutter or fibrillation in patients with history of WPW (Wolff-Parkinson-White) or LGL (Lown-Ganong-Levine) syndromes.

F. Contraindicated in patients who have known hypersensitivity.

Administration – by direct physician order only

A. *Adult* – 2.5–5.0 mg slowly IV (over 2–3 minutes). May administer additional 5–10 mg if no response in 30 minutes.

B. *Pediatric* – Not indicated for field use.

Side effects and special notes

A. Transient drop in the arterial pressure is expected. Cardiac output is usually unchanged. However, with occasional severe hypotension, treatment may be necessary. If so, the following should be considered: IV fluids, dopamine, calcium, or glucagon. Consult base physician.

B. Electrical activity through the SA and AV nodes depends to a significant degree upon calcium influx through the slow channel. By blocking that response, patients with prior nodal disease (sick sinus syndrome or second degree AV block) can develop sinus arrest, third degree heart block or asystole. These complications may require: calcium, atropine, glucagon or cardiac pacing. Consult physician.

C. Verapamil can cause severe hypotension, shock, and ventricular fibrillation when administered to a patient in ventricular tachycardia. It should not be used to differentiate PSVT from VT. When in doubt treat rhythm as ventricular tachycardia by using lidocaine.

D. Significant side effects may be rare, but life threatening. Verapamil should not be administered except where careful monitoring of vital signs and cardiac rhythm are available, with medications and defibrillation at hand to treat complications. Cardiac rhythms *must* be documented before and after the use of verapamil.

9

OPERATIONAL PROCEDURES

Operation – 1) performance of a practical work or of something involving the practical application of principles or processes.

Webster

This chapter deals with the practical issues involved in taking medical care out to the streets and homes of our communities. Interactions with various agencies and legal issues can present many challenges for the prehospital care giver. The following procedures or community decisions are examples of issues that should be addressed in any system.

COMMUNICATION PROCEDURE

Ambulance ID
A. Call number, vehicle ID.

B. Status or code – emergency, non-emergency.

C. Request physician if consultation desired.

D. Specify consultation need ("need drug orders, need hold", etc.)

E. Patients – number, age, sex.

History
A. Basic problem or chief complaint – syncope, chest pain, auto accident with neck pain, etc.

B. Pertinent additional symptoms – vomiting blood, short of breath, etc.

C. Past history *only* if pertinent – medications, similar problems in past.

Objective findings
A. General status – minor injuries, shocky, near dead, etc.

B. State of consciousness.

C. Pertinent localized findings – lacerations, broken bones, areas of tenderness, mini-neuro exam if appropriate, etc. (*only* in as much detail as necessary to prepare for the patient or to direct treatment enroute).

D. Vital signs – pulse, BP, respirations, monitor pattern if appropriate.

E. Time course since arrival – stable, gradual deterioration or improvement, etc.

Treatment
A. In progress – IVs, medications, backboards, collars, splints, etc.

B. Requests – name of attendant, specific procedure/drug request.

Estimated time of arrival

Special notes
A. Communications must be brief, orderly, precise, and void of premature or unnecessary conclusions.

B. Outstanding objective findings may take precedence over history and need to be reported first.

C. Relate medical information without using 10-codes. Direct and precise language is appreciated by all concerned.

D. Radio reports broadcast potentially confidential and privileged information. Use discretion. Patient names rarely need to be broadcast.

E. Reports should seldom take more than 1 or 2 minutes per patient. Remember your purposes: to described the problem in enough detail to explain treatment initiated and requests, and to advise the hospital of the nature and seriousness of the patient's problem so that they can be appropriately prepared for your arrival. Do not "fill" the radio report with unimportant details of history or physical. You may find that you have lost your audience by the time you get to the important information.

F. While diagnosis in the field is often not possible and personnel are cautioned against drawing inappropriate conclusions in the field, it is acceptable, and even preferable for the sake of brevity, to described a "probable hip fracture" rather than a "shortened, externally rotated leg with tenderness in the hip area".

G. The longest radio reports will usually be those where the patient is refusing care, but obviously needs care. To explain all the circumstances, what means have been tried to persuade the patients to come to the hospital, and what other attempts may be tried (including having the patient speak to the physician) will all take time. These calls are the only ones where time *should* be lengthy to try every means possible to persuade patients who may be frightened, ignorant, or even suicidal. The alternative of restraint and hauling patients against their will should be reserved for the most clearly incompetent and medically at risk patients.

PREHOSPITAL MEDICAL RECORDS (TRIP REPORT)

After the call, it is important to take the time to complete a trip report which contains all of the pertinent observations from the call. There are several reasons to accurately document observations, assessments, treatments, and patient response to treatment.

A. The first and most important reason for accurate documentation is to assure that all pertinent data has been conveyed to the receiving EMT, nurse and/or physician. This report should accompany the patient into the hospital and be available to the consultants who will ultimately provide ongoing care for the patient. Thus, it is essential to provide continuity of care. Remember, none of the in-hospital personnel will ever have access to the background information available at the scene unless it is documented in the trip report.

B. Documentation in the trip report allows CQI activities to detect problems and reveal system successes.

C. Finally, the accurate and detailed trip report can be the best defense against legal challenges regarding the medical care delivered in the field.

Hand written reports are still the most common, but more areas are investigating computer assisted reports. Certainly these are faster, more legible, and allow tremendously improved data analysis. The narrative report, however, should not be sacrificed for typing speed, poor handwriting, or fatigue. The written report must be considered almost as important as the care delivered.

The "SOAP" format is probably the most simple and widely used in medical reports. It is easy to learn and helps organize the thoughts of the prehospital care provider as well as organize the report. It also allows organization of the data in a manner consistent with hospital records, thus making interpretation by physicians and nurses easier.

"S" Subjective findings – What the patient complains of or "History".

1. Chief complaint (preferably in the patient's own words).

2. History of the present illness (When did it start? What has happened since then? What makes it better or worse? What are the associated symptoms?)

3. Past medical history *if pertinent* (History of diabetes? hypertension? heart disease?)

4. Medications (What meds are they normally taking? Any new ones? Any they *should* be on, but ran out of?)

5. Allergies (particularly drug allergies).

6. Pertinent information from family, bystanders, witnesses.

"O"   Objective findings – What you see, hear, feel, measure, or smell, on your "Physical Exam".

1. General description (awake, unconscious, comfortable, in acute respiratory distress, combative, cooperative, etc.)

2. Vital signs (blood pressure, pulse, respiratory rate.)

3. Head and neck, eyes, ears, nose, throat *if pertinent* (pupils equal or unequal, severe laceration, jugular venous distension, etc.)

4. Chest (crepitance, breath sounds, etc.)

5. Abdomen *if pertinent* (soft, tender, etc.)

6. Extremities *if pertinent* (tender, misshaped, edema, pulses, etc.)

7. Neurologic exam *if pertinent* (unconscious, response to voice, response to pain, oriented, etc.)

"A"   Assessment – What do you think is the problem?

This is not a "diagnosis", but rather an assessment of what the problem is for the patient. "Cardiac arrest" does not need a "possible" with it. It is certainly appropriate, however, to list "possible" MI or fracture.

"P"   Plan – What will you or did you do to help the patient?

Oxygen, immobilization, splinting, defibrillation, administration of medications, etc.

Record the *response* to each treatment and where the patient was transported.

Example of a prehospital medical record

S CC – Chest Pain
This 48 year old male states he developed severe "crushing" pain in his chest 2 hours ago. It has become increasingly more severe, with trouble breathing and nausea. He has had no vomiting or sweating. Wife called 911.
Past history of diabetes and hypertension.
Meds – Insulin and Inderal.
Allergic to aspirin.

O Alert and cooperative male who appears uncomfortable.
VS – BP 210/120   P 120   RR 36
HEENT – No JVD
Chest – few rales both bases
Ext – mild ankle edema

A Chest pain, probable cardiac.

P O_2 6 L/min by nasal cannula – seemed to improve respiratory distress.
Cardiac monitor – few PVCs, none significant.
IV NS, 1000 ml at TKO rate.
Nitro spray x 2 with good relief of pain.
Transport, non-emergent, Hospital X per pt choice.

CUSTOMER SERVICE

Customer service is the buzz word today. The concept of *"Do unto others as you would have them do unto you"*, however, has been around for awhile. It doesn't matter how technically adept we become if the human side of medical care is lost. Patients *expect* medical competence, but *feel better* if they are *cared for*.

The patient calling for emergency medical assistance is even more sensitive than usual. No one gets up Tuesday and writes in their day planner book – "call 911 – 7:00 P.M., Wednesday". What ever happens, it was not planned. People are not prepared – mentally, emotionally, or physically. The emergency intrusion into their day was not what they had in mind when they got up this morning. This makes the prehospital care provider's approach, *attitude*, dress, and manners critical to the interaction.

Essential elements of patient oriented "customer" care (may seem similar to scouting):

1. Be prompt.

2. Be neat, clean, courteous.

3. Address patient and family by last names if possible, "Mr or Mrs Jones", *not* "Joe" or "Sally". (First name only if patient requests.)

4. Address patients and family by "sir" or "madam" if unable to obtain or remember names or in critical patient situations.

5. Be courteous and appropriate with other personnel. It is inappropriate to bicker with or put down other prehospital care providers in front of patient or family. If you have a problem with paramedic X or police officer Y – address it *after* the call. If you have recurring problems, ask a supervisor's assistance, but reach an agreement about how you will handle problems at the scene with this other person *before* the next call. (They should be motivated to reach an agreement, since you are not making their job easier, either.)

6. Be neat at the scene. Do not leave bloody needles, wraps, tape or bandages, etc., lying around. It used to be sloppy, but in the time of AIDS and hepatitis, it is also dangerous.

7. Be considerate of patient comfort. If there is no life threat then take the time to make the patient as comfortable as possible. Are they

worried about their dog? Confine him and reassure patient. Are they worried about friends or neighbors? Advise those on the scene where the patient will be transported. Are they cold? or in pain? Get another blanket or call in for pain medication. There may be reasons *not* to medicate in the field, but there are at least as many times that it *is* indicated. Call and confer with the physician.

8. Be considerate of family and friends. Advise them where patient will be transported and whether that will be emergent or non-emergent. (Families are often outraged when they arrive at the hospital before the ambulance. They *assume* that the ambulance will go faster – in fact they often assume that is why they should call an ambulance. When the time is available, explain how the patient will be transported and *why*.)

9. Be considerate of the patient. You will have time during the majority of non-emergent runs to explain what all of the menacing looking equipment is. You may explain what you are doing. On a "routine" run, ask how the patient feels about his day being interrupted. Ask how you can make him more comfortable.

10. Be considerate and professional at the hospital. Give a complete patient report. If the physician or nurse seem distracted – ask if you should give the report after they have the patient settled. Sometimes you can avoid being asked dozens of questions if you wait until the hospital staff can give you their full attention.

11. Try to anticipate for the patient what will happen in the hospital, but not predict exact tests or disposition.

12. Treat the patient as you would wish to be treated if you were the patient.

HEALTH/WELLNESS/FITNESS/BURNOUT

Prehospital care providers need to be reminded and encouraged to *look out for number one.*

All care providers are at risk for "burnout". The definition of this term varies, but most people recognize the provider who must quit, because they have nothing more to "provide". There is a very real risk for personnel in "giving" or "helper" professions. They are so busy giving care to others they forget to care for themselves.

Rx for health and wellness:

A. Make time for family. Your spouse and children may seem the biggest drain on your time, but they will also be the biggest, most effective support system you can develop. There is no other use of your time that will provide as many short and long term rewards. There will be only limited opportunities to participate in those critical times in your children's lives. Whether it's the dance recital, the big wrestling match, the first concert, or the big debate, you can't make them all. The critical ones your spouse will point out, your children will point out, and you had best listen! Change your schedule, trade a shift or get someone to cover you. Those moments are rare and will enrich your life.

Your spouse or significant other will participate in your stressful life at some level, (your stress will be passed on to them) so make time to talk and plan and enjoy each other with some activities just for the two of you. Those times also will seem rare but precious, and can keep the relationship alive.

If you don't have a spouse or significant other – get a pet! Everyone needs someone at home to talk to and play with. Dogs and cats are certainly the most popular. There is some experimental data that retirement home residents do better and live longer with pets. Children in hospitals may heal faster with pets. They are certainly less demanding than spouses, and don't care *how late* you get home. Very beneficial for those who haven't found Mr or Ms Right!

B. Eat well. Living in the rig (or in a fire station) is no excuse to live on potato chips and soda or ice cream and fat. Even 7-11 now offers fresh fruits and lower fat, nongreasy sandwiches. Bag lunches are still a very good way to get good nutrition if you use

341

your imagination and creativity to avoid the peanut butter and jelly or bologna routine. OSHA regulations prohibit eating in the ambulance, but the radio should still alert you if you are at a roadside park. If you are eating with a group you must make the extra effort to educate your co-workers that healthful food can still be very tasty. Low fat, low cholesterol diets should be the rule with complex carbohydrates, fresh fruits and vegetables making up the bulk of your diet. This doesn't mean those banana splits will disappear forever, but make the treats just that . . . infrequent, *and just for a treat.*

C. Manage stress. Most of you are stress seekers. Your job is concentrated stress. Some of that is good. It keeps us interested and mentally active. Too much, however, without "management" leads to fatigue, disinterest and "burnout". Find your own personal method of stress management. It is not the same for everyone. Consider which of the following may help your stress – and incorporate that regularly in your weekly schedule.

1. Exercise. Always incorporate this one . . . it's the only one that works for everyone. This can be long walks, jogging, swimming, bicycling, or mountain climbing, but assure some type of aerobic exercise routine in your life. Tennis, racquetball, baseball, football, golf or other sports should be included only if they are *fun*. If you have to *win* at tennis it will add to the stress, not reduce it.

2. Music. Whether it is listening, singing or playing an instrument, music soothes not only the beast, but also the rest of us.

3. Meditation. Significant data are available to indicate humans can have tremendous control over their blood pressure and pulse with meditation. If it works for you – do it.

4. Hobbies. If you can lose the immediate problems of the world by immersing yourself in a collection or project – this may be for you. Consider woodworking, sewing, knitting, gardening or other activities that provide a peaceful alternative to your stress side.

5. Movies or plays. Another chance to "escape" to another world and leave the tension behind.

6. Biofeedback. As with meditation, this has some good data to recommend it, but you be the final judge if it works for you.

7. Massage. Therapeutic massage is a good way to reward yourself for working hard. When provided by your spouse or significant other it can lead to other very important stress reducing activities.

8. Laugh. Don't take yourself too seriously. Humor has been a classic stress reducer for eons. Keep some of your favorite funny stories to pass on to your colleagues. You needn't laugh at patients or friends. Yet you can still laugh at the situations in which they find themselves involved.

D. Exercise. Again, this is the easiest and most important thing you can do to improve health and reduce stress. Regular aerobic exercise is the most effective way to achieve physical fitness. This can reduce blood pressure, reduce resting pulse, and lower adrenergic tone. As you improve your cardiovascular fitness, you will have more energy, less fatigue, and increased ability to deal with stress.

E. Stop smoking. If you get enough exercise, you won't be able to smoke. Find what your personal excuses are, and find a way around them.

F. Drinking. Be careful. Small amounts can be a stress reducer, but effects are short lived and it is too tempting to return to the bottle in response to stress. Cautious and responsible alcohol ingestion can be a pleasant addition to meals and social events.

PROFESSIONAL IDENTITY

There has been some debate recently as to whether prehospital care work is an occupation or a profession. There are many EMTs and Paramedics, however, who are too busy studying, training, or providing patient care to enter the debate. In many cases these are the professionals who set the standards others are trying to achieve. Webster defines profession as "1 - a professing, or declaring; avowal 2 - an occupation requiring advanced academic training. . . ". Perhaps it rests with the individual. Just as the "professional" actor or writer is distinguished from the person who is "just doing their job", the paramedic who sets the example and participates at all levels is the one thought of as a "professional."

The professional frequently excels within their own employment environment. They are the supervisors, field internship evaluators, infection disease officers, or CQI consultants for their efforts. They are frequently the ones going to conferences, bringing back new ideas, and constantly asking why or why not. (This does not always make them the favorites of management – even if we would like to think it should.)

The professionals participate on a state and national level with organizations representing their field. The National Association of Emergency Medical Technicians (NAEMT) is an organization that represent the interests of the EMT and Paramedic. There are also state component organizations.

NAEMT

The National Association of Emergency Medical Technicians was founded in 1975. It was established to be the national voice for EMT and Paramedic professionals.

In the 20 years since that foundation it has alternated between strength and weakness – growth or implosion – but it has remained the only national voice of the prehospital care professional. Its national membership has become a strength in training, public education, and discussions of health system reform.

NAEMT represents over 400,000 EMTs working across the U.S. and gives voice to their professional concerns and interests.

NAEMT was instrumental in obtaining Public Safety Officers Benefits for EMTs as well as police officers and firefighters.

NAEMT has been active in developing and supporting a wide variety of educational workshops and programs. These range from the annual meetings which host thousands of EMTs and hundreds of companies demonstrating their prehospital equipment to small intensive learning experiences such as the Prehospital Trauma Life Support (PHTLS) courses.

Membership includes voting for state representatives to represent local interests at the national level. It includes a newsletter which contains current issues and educational events. It also includes a subscription to the *Journal of Emergency Medical Services* at a reduced rate. *JEMS* magazine is one of the most informative publications with the widest range of interests and topics – always on the "cutting edge".

Professionals strive to challenge themselves and to be the best they can be. Many will take the National Registry of Emergency Medical Technicians (NREMT) exam and maintain registration, even if it is not mandatory for their particular job. The National Registry exam and continuing education requirements are currently the best assurance to the public that an EMT or Paramedic is a quality care provider.

NREMT

In 1969 President Lyndon Johnson's Committee on Highway Traffic Safety recommended that there be a national certification agency to establish uniform standards for training and examination of personnel active in the delivery of emergency ambulance service. A task force was formed that year and the National Registry of Emergency Medical Technicians had its first formal meeting in 1970. The Board of Directors was composed of representatives of the Ambulance Association of America (later to become the American Ambulance Association), International Association of Fire Chiefs, International Rescue and First Aid Association, National Ambulance and Medical Services Association, National Funeral Directors Association, National Sheriffs Association, and International Association of Chiefs of Police. These seven organizational members nominated four physicians involved in EMS to join the Board as it was established as an independent, not-for-profit, non-governmental, free-standing agency.

The first basic NREMT-A examination was administered simultaneously to 1,520 ambulance personnel at 51 test sites throughout the United States in October, 1971. Reregistration guidelines were developed for the EMT-Ambulance and the "EMT-Non Ambulance" in 1975. The development of a national training program for EMT-Paramedic lead to new paramedic exams being written in 1977. The development of guidelines and examinations for the EMT-Intermediate level was completed in 1980. Continued work since then has expanded the question bases while maintaining currency of the exam as medical practice standards have changed. NREMT has also been very involved in the development of the field of prehospital practice on the national level. They have participated with the Joint Review Committee for EMT-Paramedic Education since its inception with the AMA. Most recently they sponsored the National EMS Education and Practice Blueprint. This project will directly impact the EMT-Basic update as well as updates for the other levels of prehospital care providers.

National Registration is dependent on passing both a written and practical exam. The written exam is developed in stages. The item writing committee is formed with prehospital personnel, EMS experts, and educators from across the country invited to develop questions over certain course objectives. These must all be referenced to assigned objectives with answers available in commonly used EMT textbooks. The committee then meets to review, rewrite and reconstruct drafted items. Consensus by the committee must be gained so that each question is in direct reference to the curriculum, that the correct answer is the one and only correct answer, that each distractor option has some plausibility, and the answer can be found within commonly available EMT textbooks. Controversial questions are discarded and not placed within the item banks. Items are reviewed for reading level and to ensure that no bias exists related to race, gender, or ethnicity.

Following completion of the item writing phase, all items are then pilot tested in areas across the United States. Item analysis is completed. A Standard Setting Committee then meets to determine the pass/fail score of the examination using a criterion-referenced technique as guided by psychometric consultants. Members of the Standard Setting Committee are expert in prehospital care and may include EMT-Basics, Intermediates, Paramedics, Nurse-Paramedics, State EMS Directors, State Training Coordinators or Physicians. All members of the committee review every portion of a test item including the stem, correct answer and distractors. All members must agree on the construction of the question and affirm the correctly keyed answer. Following the modified Nedelsky formula, a performance index is determined for each item in the National Registry's item bank. Examinations are then developed based upon an analysis of the most frequent and critical tasks EMTs perform when providing prehospital care. All examinations are constructed to have a pass/fail standard of 70%.

The practical examination is currently based on published standards. If those standards are learned and *practiced* it would be difficult not to pass the practical exam. Maintenance of registration is dependent on continuing education. These standards were originally based on a "best guess" from many experts in the field, but are constantly being challenged both from within and without the Registry. There is currently planned a research project to address the issue of continuing education needs for prehospital care personnel. The issue is very difficult to sort out, as conflicting data from other medical care areas indicate.

In spite of controversy over the *amount* of continuing education necessary, there does not seem to be any disagreement that on-going education is necessary for *all* fields of medical care. National Registration, then, remains the best assurance to the public of a quality prehospital care provider.

So, is it a profession? *The choice is yours.*

INFECTIOUS DISEASES

Infectious diseases have been of increased concern for prehospital care workers over the past several years. The impetus for this concern is the Acquired Immune Deficiency Syndrome, but it has been recognized for some time that prehospital care workers were at increased risk for Hepatitis B, Meningitis, Tuberculosis, and other more rare conditions. Since there is no way of determining which of the patients will have underlying infectious diseases, the current recommendations are for "Universal Body Substance Precautions". This includes protecting the prehospital care worker from specific exposure to patient blood, urine, feces, saliva, etc. Routine use of good hand washing technique, and proper cleansing of equipment will help decrease the risk of contamination.

Summary of Current Recommendations:

1. Immunization

    a. MMR - measles, mumps, and rubella

    b. Polio

    c. DPT or DT - diphtheria, pertussis, and tetanus

    d. Heptavax or Recombivax - Hepatitis B

    e. Influenza (optional, but desirable)

2. Gloves should be worn for all anticipated exposure to body fluids. At a minimum this includes all trauma patients, all intravenous lines, any patient who is incontinent or markedly disheveled.

3. Goggles or glasses should be worn for any anticipated splattering exposure. Masks are also recommended when possible. This particularly applies to patients needing intubation. OSHA *requires* use of goggles *and* masks if splatter can be "reasonably anticipated".

4. If unanticipated contact with any body substance occurs – washing should be performed as soon as possible (hands, face, etc.). Contaminated clothing should be removed as soon as possible and washed with chlorine bleach before reuse.

5. If exposure to a patient's body fluids has occurred the receiving emergency physician should be notified. A routine mechanism

must exist to notify the Infection Control Officer of each organization who can review details of exposure, and patient status and determine whether HIV, Hepatitis B, or other tests are necessary for the prehospital care worker. Follow-up recommendations may be from a company or "Work Comp" physician, from the physician adviser or other infection control physician associated with the organization. It is very important that the details of the paper work and information flow be established before the events occur. Certainly exposures will continue to occur (though, hopefully, less often), and the Ryan White Act has dictated many of the informational steps that will occur if the hospital becomes aware of a patient with a communicable disease who may have exposed a prehospital care worker to that disease.

6. In the event of *significant* exposure (deep puncture wound) to *known* HIV + patient, the prehospital care worker should be evaluated *immediately* (checked in as an emergency department patient if that is the only alternative on nights, weekends, etc.). The prehospital care worker should be evaluated, the risks assessed and they should be offered AZT if appropriate (and after receiving full information on the advantages and disadvantages of that drug or any alternative).

INTERHOSPITAL TRANSFER

Interhospital patient transfers on an emergency basis are commonly initiated when definitive diagnostic or therapeutic needs of a patient are beyond the capacity of one hospital. The patient is potentially unstable and medical treatment must be continued and possibly even initiated enroute. Written guidelines permit orderly transfer of patients with appropriate continuity of care. COBRA has mandated such policies be established by each hospital. The following is a suggested protocol:

A. All patients should be stabilized as much as possible before transfer.

B. Paramedics or EMTs must receive an adequate summary of the patient's condition, current treatment, possible complications and other pertinent medical information.

C. Treatment orders should be given to the ambulance personnel. These orders should be in writing. Orders given by direct verbal order from the doctor who is initiating the transfer must be recorded immediately, and signed prior to transport.

D. Any patient sick enough for emergency transfer must have at least one IV in place prior to transfer. Orders for IV composition and rate should be provided.

E. Transfer papers (summary, lab work, X-rays, etc.) should be given to the ambulance personnel, not to the family or friends.

F. The receiving physician must be contacted by the transferring physician prior to transfer. The base physician may also need to be contacted so that appropriate radio control of the ambulance enroute is assured.

G. The receiving hospital, physician, and nursing personnel must be notified prior to initiation of transfer to assure adequate space and the ability to care for this patient.

H. The personnel and equipment used to transfer a patient should be appropriate to the treatment needed or anticipated during transfer. EMTs who are not familiar with IVs should not handle emergency transfers. Paramedics should be utilized if any advanced resuscitation or treatment is anticipated. In specialized fields not ordinarily handled by paramedics (e.g., obstetrics, high risk newborns), appropriately trained personnel (e.g., nurse, physician and/or respiratory therapist) should accompany the patient.

In order to maintain these standards, it may be appropriate for the receiving hospital to send an ambulance with more specifically trained personnel to transfer the patient. This is particularly true in the case of newborns, but has also been shown to be effective in other critically ill or injured patients.

LEGAL PROBLEMS

State laws which govern emergency medical care vary. Legal problems which develop during an emergency call are best managed by direct communication between the providers and the base physician, or, ideally, between the patient and the physician. The following is an outline of basic legal principles which may be useful when no direct contact with base physician is possible.

Consent

A. A mentally competent patient has the right to consent to or to refuse treatment. If the patient is not mentally competent, a competent relative or guardian has this same right (see below).

B. Consent is "implied" when the patient is unable to consent to treatment due to age, mental status or medical condition and no responsible party is available to grant that consent.

C. *In no event should legal consent procedures be allowed to delay immediately required treatment.* If the time delay to obtain lawful consent from an authorized person would present a serious risk of death or serious impairment of health, or would prolong severe pain or suffering of the patient, treatment may be undertaken to avoid that risk.

D. Age of consent varies with different states. In general, the patient must be over 18 years of age or between 15 and 18 years and "emancipated", (i.e., living apart from his or her parents).

E. If the patient is a minor, consent should be from a competent natural parent, adopted parent, or legal guardian.

Mental Competence

A. A person is mentally competent if he or she:

1. is able to understand the nature and consequences of his or her illness or injury,

2. is able to understand the nature and consequences of the proposed treatment, and

3. has sufficient emotional control, judgment, and discretion to manage his or her own affairs.

   The patient should be assessed to determine that they are

oriented, have an understanding of what happened, and what may possibly happen if treated or not treated, and have a plan of action – such as how to get home from scene if refusing treatment.

B. A patient who is intoxicated, under the influence of drugs or toxic inhalation (CO poisoning), head injured, or in shock will most likely *not* be considered competent.

C. If the patient is not mentally competent under these guidelines, consent should be obtained from another responsible party – who must also be mentally competent and legally "of age": spouse, adult son or daughter, parent, adult brother or sister, or legal guardian.

D. If the patient is not mentally competent and none of the above persons can be reached, the person should be treated and transported to a medical facility. It is preferable to enlist support and agreement in this course of action from a police officer.

Duty to Act
A. Public and municipal ambulances have a duty to respond to all calls for aid in their response area and to render appropriate treatment. (Private services may be immune from this requirement. Volunteer no-pay services may have this duty to respond also.)

B. The prehospital provider has an obligation to treat the patient in accordance with the standard of care to be expected from other medical care providers of the same training and skill level. If the responder does not act in accordance with those accepted standards of care *and* the patient suffers injury because of this, the provider may be liable for negligence.

C. Once treatment has been rendered, the prehospital provider has the duty to care for that patient until he can transfer care to a competent health care provider who accepts responsibility for the patient (either at the scene, en route, or in the hospital).

Special Notes
A. Failure to treat someone who needs care is a far "riskier" course than to treat in good faith with less than full legal permission.

Do not let fear of legal consequences keep you from rendering such responsible and competent care as your patient has a right to expect from your medical training.

B. The best defense against any legal question of consent, competence, and the need for care, is a good *medical record*. Your written account of the patient and care rendered will be invaluable to you if legal questions are raised months later and will convey your competence and adherence to standards of care.

COMMUNITY DECISIONS

The following situations should be discussed at length is each community whether at the County Medical Society, EMS council, or whatever organization is involved and responsible for EMS activities. As noted previously, the discussion should begin with what level of prehospital care each community desires, what level they can support, and what resources are available. Since the emergency physicians are also frequently the individuals involved in the training and direction of the prehospital care personnel, they must be involved in the discussions from the outset. Discussion should then continue to equipment needed or wanted and drugs to be carried. The community physicians should be involved in discussions to determine what interventions will be acceptable to the community. The emergency physicians particularly, will need to determine what field direction they will be comfortable providing on the radio. Once the pieces are in place the system needs "fine-tuning". Radio reports, written trip reports, and similar guidelines are included earlier in this chapter. The following issues, however, are very dependent on the local community and must be discussed.

How will your community deal with the following:

Patient refusals

If a call has been placed for assistance and a patient has been contacted at a scene and he refuses to be transported, this is a refusal. These patients should be appropriately assessed, including taking vital signs. The condition of the patient must be documented. If this is not possible, the reason should be described on the trip report. All refusals may be called in to base hospital via a med channel or a recorded line. This will provide an opportunity for the base physician to discuss with the prehospital personnel what the situation is and whether the physician can persuade a patient who needs care to come to the hospital. Many times a physician (even by radio) can make the difference in the patient's decision to seek medical care. This also allows a recording to be made of the discussion and specifically, how many ways were tried to persuade someone who needs care to come to the hospital. For those infrequent, but legally terrifying cases, when the patient becomes worse, or dies, it is invaluable to have a recording of the fact that prehospital personnel advised patient to go to hospital and advised of possible complications, including death if patient continued to refuse transport. These recordings may be available for a varying period of time. Most can be made available for an indefinite period if there are any potential legal problems. This policy is for the protection of the prehospital care worker, as well as the patient. Many problems can be avoided by involving the base physician in the discussion as soon as a potential problem is recognized.

Prehospital care workers are also encouraged to document that refusal was called in by writing on the trip report, "Hospital (specify name) notified of refusal" or "Dr. X at Hospital Y approved refusal" if there is any conflict. As with medications, the prehospital personnel are advised to request a physician on the radio immediately if there is a concern with a refusal.

Refusals fall into the following variety of situations:

1. If the patient and the EMT or paramedic agree no medical problem exists and no treatment is necessary, then no transport is needed. Call in refusal, but no need to speak with physician. This may be recorded by the nurse if they are also comfortable with the refusal.

2. If the EMT or paramedic feels no medical problem exists and no treatment is necessary and the patient feels he *does* need care and wishes transportation, the patient should be transported or medical control consulted. Many systems have variable policies in this regard local protocols must be developed.

3. If the EMT or paramedic believes the patient needs medical care and the patient does not agree, the prehospital worker must decide if the patient is competent to make that decision.

    a. If the patient is alert, oriented and understands the need for treatment and the possible consequences of not receiving treatment – he may refuse treatment. The EMT or paramedic should document this on the trip report and by radio communication with an emergency physician at the base hospital.

    b. If the EMT or paramedic has determined the patient is not competent to understand the need for treatment and/or the risks of refusal, the patient may be transported without his consent. (Consider this if the patient appears to have a head injury, significant alcohol intake, altered mental status, abnormal vital signs, or any chemical contamination that may have produced less than optimal brain function.) This must also be well documented. Some areas have a medical or psychiatric "hold" that will assist with confining patients until they are mentally capable of caring for themselves. Some areas have judges on call to make these decisions.

4. Children (below age 18) are not competent legally to make medical care decisions. If care is needed – transport with parents agreement. If care is needed – and no parents or relatives are available – transport and parents will be notified by the hospital. If care is needed – and parents refuse – notify legal authorities who can place the child in protective custody for medical care. If no care is needed – child *must* be left with a competent adult. Older children may appropriately be left in their own care, but consult with base physician. Call in refusal.

5. Prehospital care personnel need to be reassured that when in doubt, base hospital emergency physician should be consulted. These are frequently time consuming and emotionally trying cases, but have the greatest medical and legal risks. They are worth discussion in advance and sometimes prolonged discussions when they occur.

Another challenging prehospital occurrence:

Physician on scene

Physician and paramedic interactions can be very positive or very negative, but they are seldom boring exchanges. These interactions will occur under different circumstances and the rules will change with the circumstances.

A. Physicians with critical patients in their office (or other facility) call for help and transport. The prehospital care provider will be going into the personal office or facility of the physician to attend the physician's patient. The physician caring for the patient has been in charge of events to that point in time and frequently will be somewhat reluctant to "turn over" that charge position. On the other hand they are also frequently quite anxious to get the patient out of their facility, so they may seem quite torn by this dilemma. The easier the prehospital personnel make this transition, the better it will go. Paramedics are encouraged to get as much of the history as possible while actually loading the patient. IV access may already be accomplished or may need to be performed at the scene or enroute. If the physician is anxious to get the patient out, the "Load and Go" mentality may be evident. If that is the case IV access can be established enroute.

If the patient is in cardiac arrest, the initial approach will need to be accomplished in the physician's office. This will probably be the most difficult situation to accomplish smoothly. Most physicians will not be able to just "stand back" and let the prehospital personnel run a cardiac arrest in their office. If the physician is helpful – paramedics are encouraged to let them help! If the physician is interrupting procedures, demanding drugs not carried, or otherwise obstructing the scene – the base physician may need to be consulted to assist with the physician communication needs (hand the radio to the on scene physician). If necessary, the patient will need to be transported with procedures performed enroute. That attending physician will be considered legally in charge of *their* patient in *their* facility.

B. The physician who "stops by" at the scene is in the role of a "Good Samaritan". They have no established relationship with this patient (unless they advise you otherwise). These physicians also, may be of great assistance or great annoyance. *Some of their attitude can come from the prehospital care providers!* When treated with respect and asked for specific assistance they will most likely be quite helpful. If there is a confrontation, however, their position is weaker than the physician in his own office. Most likely this physician has no legal authority on the scene. If this is an auto accident or other public incident the scene commander will be spelled out in city/ county statutes . . . and it will not be a physician. If necessary, the physician can be forcefully removed from the scene, but someone's diplomacy rating must be quite low to ever get to that level of action. Paramedics are encouraged to try instead, to utilize the physician's assistance in productive ways.

C. Some Medical Societies have directed that a physician wishing to take responsibility for a patient on the scene "must identify him/herself as a physician and should be able to show his license; otherwise paramedics are obligated to continue their treatment of the patient". *If the physician assumes responsibility for the patient, it is his/her responsibility to stay with that patient until reaching the hospital, preferably in the transporting vehicle.* If a physician on scene insists on assuming care, their license can be requested and they can be requested to sign a form accepting responsibility (next page). The legal principles would sway between a physician, who may be supposed to be better capable of rendering emergency patient care, and a paramedic who may be legally in charge of the scene (refer to specific county/city ordinances). It is always prudent to avoid these patient conflicts, but they do occur and are better handled if thought out and discussed in advance.

A final essential topic for community consideration:

Futile care

A. Many systems are writing guidelines to determine which patients can be allowed to die at home and which need evaluation and care in a hospital. Many areas of the country are wrestling with DNR legislation and to whom it applies. Many patients are demanding a louder voice in their own care. Patients with chronic disease are deciding whether they wish to live with a tube in their airway. The answers are not always what the medical establishment expects. All of these situations require thoughtful consideration by the physicians and personnel involved in establishing the prehospital care system. The discussions should include ethicists as well as lay personnel.

B. How much is *enough* and how much is *too much*? Consider guidelines that will allow the paramedics to *stop* work on patients who are unresponsive to usual resuscitation measures. Some general guidelines are included in "Death in the Field" and "Special Trauma Problems", but many other situations exist that are not appropriate for transport. The hiker who fell 20 feet, is in cardiopulmonary arrest, and requires a 2 hour extrication, will probably not be worked on, but there are an equal number of equally unsalvageable patients who do receive CPR in this country. Additional research may need to be performed for some areas, but many areas could improve their system just by getting the correct people sitting around the table and discussing alternatives.

And with these attempts to make prehospital care more appropriate for the living and the dead, don't forget the prehospital care personnel who will be making those decisions. They need to be involved in the discussions before guidelines are written, and involved in critiques later. Additional training may be needed to make them more comfortable with the new problems created when they are left with a live family and a dead patient. It suddenly seems much easier to start CPR and transport . . . no family to deal with, nothing that must be said, no searching for the right words, just load and go and do what they are trained to do. They *must* receive some additional training before they take on the additional roles. There are benefits, however, to a prehospital system that is as expert at providing comfort to grieving relatives, as to inserting tubes in gasping airways.

PHYSICIAN RESPONSIBILITY AT THE SCENE

A physician wishing to take responsibility for a patient on the scene must identify him/herself as a physician and should be able to show his license; otherwise, paramedics are obligated to continue their treatment of the patient. *If the physician assumes responsibility for the patient, it is his/her responsibility to stay with that patient until reaching the hospital, preferably in the transporting vehicle.*

As a physician who plans to assume care of this patient, I understand that the paramedics are acting under standing orders and are performing under the license of their medical director. I feel that I can provide care to this patient which is more beneficial than that available through the prehospital care system of EMTs and Paramedics. I request, therefore that I be allowed to assume care and I agree to accompany the patient to the hospital.

_____

Signature

_____

Please print name

Tear this form out and transport with the patient to the hospital.

Abbreviation Key

ABC = airway, breathing, circulation
ACEP = American College of Emergency Physicians
ACLS = Advanced Cardiac Life Support
ACS = American College of Surgeons
ALS = Advanced Life Support
AOB = odor of alcohol on breath
ATLS = Advanced Trauma Life Support

BTLS = Basic Trauma Life Support
BLS = Basic Life Support
BP = blood pressure
BVM = bag-valve-mask

C = Centigrade
CC = chief complaint
CCU = coronary care unit
CHF = congestive heart failure
CNS = central nervous system
CO = carbon monoxide
CO_2 = carbon dioxide
COPD = chronic obstructive pulmonary disease
CPR = cardiopulmonary resuscitation

CQI = continuous quality improvement
CSF = cerebrospinal fluid
CSM = carotid sinus massage
C-spine = cervical spine
CVA = cerebrovascular accident (stroke)

DOT = (U.S.) Department of Transportation
D5W = dextrose 5% in water

ED = Emergency Department
EGTA = esophageal obturator-gastric tube airway
EKG = electrocardiogram
EMD = electromechanical dissociation
EMS = Emergency Medical Services
EMT-B = Emergency Medical Technician, Basic
EMT-I = Intermediate Emergency Medical Technician
      (by DOT standards)
EMT-P = paramedic, or Emergency Medical Technician-Paramedic
EOA = esophageal obturator airway
ET tube = endotracheal tube
ETA = estimated time of arrival

F = Fahrenheit

g = gauge (diameter)
GCS = Glasgow Coma Scale or Score
gm = gram
GSW = gunshot wound
gtts = drops

HMRT = Hazardous Materials Response Team
Haz-Mat = Hazardous materials

I.C.S.= Incident Command System
ICS = intercostal space
IV = intravenous
IM = intramuscular
IO = intraosseous

J = Joule

L = liter
LMP = last menstrual period
LOC = loss of consciousness

MAST = medical anti-shock trouser
MCL = mid-clavicular line
mcg = microgram
meds = medications
mEq = milli-equivalent
mg = milligram
MI = myocardial infarction
min = minute
ml = milliliter
MS = morphine sulfate

NAEMSP = National Association of EMS Physicians
NAEMT = National Association of Emergency Medical Technicians
NG tube = nasogastric tube
NPO = nothing by mouth
NREMT = National Registry of Emergency Medical Technicians
NS = normal saline
NSR = normal sinus rhythm
NTG = nitroglycerin

O_2 = oxygen
OB = obstetrical
OD = overdose

P = pulse
PAC = premature atrial contraction
PALS = Pediatric Advanced Life Support
PASG = pneumatic anti-shock garment
PCC = Poison Control Center
PE = pulmonary edema or pulmonary embolus
PEA = pulseless electrical activity
PHTLS = Prehospital Trauma Life Support
PSVT = paroxysmal supraventricular tachycardia
PTV = percutaneous transtracheal ventilation
PVC = premature ventricular contraction

RL = ringer's lactate
RLQ = right lower quadrant
RR = respiratory rate
RUQ = right upper quadrant

sec = second
SL = sublingual
SOB = shortness of breath
SQ = subcutaneous
soln = solution
synch = synchronous (switch on defibrillator)

TIA = transient ischemic attack
TKO = to keep open (minimum IV rate)

v. fib. = ventricular fibrillation
v. tach. = ventricular tachycardia
VS = vital signs

WNL = within normal limits
W-sec = watt-second (joules)

Recommended Basic Library

1. AMA Division of Drugs & Toxicology. *AMA Drug Evaluations Annual.* American Medical Association, Chicago, 1994.

2. American Academy of Orthopedic Surgeons. *Emergency Care and Transportation of the Sick and Injured.* ed. 5 (revised). A.A.O.S., Chicago, 1993.

3. American College of Surgeons, Committee on Trauma. *Advanced Trauma Life Support Course Text.* A.C.S., 1992.

4. American Heart Association. *Textbook of Advanced Cardiac Life Support.* A.H.A., Dallas, 1994.

5. American Heart Association. *Textbook of Pediatric Advanced Life Support.* A.H.A., Dallas, 1994.

6. Barkin, R. M., and Rosen, P. *Emergency Pediatrics.* ed. 4. C. V. Mosby Co., 1994.

7. Bronstein, A.C. and Currance, P.L. *Emergency Care for Hazardous Materials Exposure.* C.V. Mosby Co., St Louis, 1988.

8. Butman, A.M., Martin, S.W., Vomacka, R.W., McSwain, N.E. *Comprehensive Guide to Pre-hospital Skills.* Emergency Training, Akron, Ohio, 1995.

9. Campbell, J. E. (ed.). *Basic Trauma Life Support for Paramedics and Advanced EMS Providers.* ed. 3. Prentice Hall, Inc., Englewood Cliffs, N.J., 1995.

10. Caroline, N. L. *Ambulance Calls: Review Problems for the Paramedic.* ed. 3. Little, Brown and Co., Boston, 1991.

11. Caroline, N. L. *Emergency Care in the Streets.* ed. 5. Little Brown and Co., Boston, 1995.

12. Department of Transportation *Emergency Response Guidebook.* US DOT Materials Transportation Bureau, Washington, DC, 1993.

13. Fitch, J.J. *Beyond the Street, A Handbook for EMS Leadership and Management.* JEMS Publishing Co., Inc., Solana Beach, CA., 1988.

14. Fleisher, G. and Ludwig, S. (eds.). *Textbook of Pediatric Emergency Medicine.* ed. 3. Williams & Wilkins, Baltimore, 1993.

15. Frew, S.A. *Street Law, Rights and Responsibilities of the EMT.* Reston Publishing Co., Virginia, 1983.

16. Gazzaniga, A. B., Iseri, L. T., and Baren, M. (eds.). *Emergency Care Principles and Practices for the EMT-Paramedic.* ed. 2. Reston Publishing, Virginia, 1982.

17. Grant, H., et. al. *Emergency Care.* ed. 7. Prentice-Hall, Inc., Englewood Cliffs, N.J., 1995.

18. Grant, H. *Vehicle Rescue.* R. J. Brady Co., Maryland, 1975.

19. Jacobs, L., and Bennett, B. R. *Emergency Patient Care: Prehospital Ground and Air Procedures.* Macmillan Publishing, New York, 1983.

20. Jones, S.A., et. al. (eds.). *Advanced Emergency Care for Paramedic Practice.* J.B. Lippincott Co., Philadelphia, 1992.

21. National Association of Emergency Medical Technicians, Prehospital Trauma Life Support Committee. *Prehospital Trauma Life Support.* Mosby-Year Book, Inc., St. Louis, 1994.

22. Newkirk, W. L. and Linden, R.P. *Managing Emergency Medical Services.* Reston Publishing Co., Virginia, 1984.

23. Rosen, P., et. al. (eds.). *Emergency Medicine: Concepts and Clinical Practice.* ed. 3. Mosby Year Book, St. Louis, 1992.

24. Sanders, M. J. *Mosby's Paramedic Textbook.* Mosby-Year Book, Inc., St. Louis, 1994.

25. Schwartz, G. R., et. al. (eds.) *Principles and Practices of Emergency Medicine.* ed. 3. Prentice Hall, Inc., Englewood Cliffs, N.J., 1992.

26. Stutz, D.R. and Ulin, S. *Hazardous Materials Injuries.* ed. 3. Bradford Communications Corporation, Maryland, 1992.

27. Walraven, G., et. al. (eds.) *Manual of Advanced Prehospital Care.* R. J. Brady, Maryland, 1984.

28. Wasserberger, J., and Eubanks, D. H. *Advanced Paramedic Procedures: A Practical Approach,* ed. 2, C. V. Mosby, St. Louis, 1983.